D0532437

...Ɔ HANDBOOK.

COMPILED BY

TOM TYLER

'TRICIA TYLER.

JACK OF ALL TRADES PUBLISHING.

WRITTEN, PRINTED AND PUBLISHED IN ENGLAND.
2012.

A CANCER PATIENTS HANDBOOK.

ISBN 978-0-9567463-1-3.

DEDICATED TO ALL CANCER PATIENTS, IN THE HOPE THAT THIS SMALL BOOK MAY BE A HELP TO THEM IN THEIR BATTLE.

PUBLISHED BY JACK OF ALL TRADES PUBLISHING, PRINTED IN ENGLAND BY THE LAVENHAM PRESS, ARBONS HOUSE, 47 WATER STREET, LAVENHAM, SUFFOLK. U.K. CO10 9RN.

Cover design and drawings by Tom Tyler.

CONTENTS

FORWARD BY Dr. CHRISTOPHER SCRASE.

Most of us will know someone who has, or who has had, cancer. It may be someone in our family, even one of our pets, our work colleagues, our neighbours or just someone we've met in passing. Each has a story to tell of their experience of that encounter with what for many is still a dreaded disease. Healthcare professionals will do their utmost to allay those anxieties, those uncertainties and those challenges.

Yet sometimes patients or their families are still left wondering what it will really *feel* like. This may not relate to the delivery of treatment, but rather the more mundane issues that so often we take for granted until our lives become disrupted by cancer.

Tom and 'Tricia have been able to articulate with great ease and comfort what it does *feel* like personally to experience the illness, and offer valued direction on how to deal with the plethora of issues that surface as a consequence. Their fascinating insight offers reassurance that it really is possible to live through and beyond this illness.

Dr. Christopher D. Scrase,
Trust Clinical Cancer Lead,
Ipswich Hospital NHS Trust. January 2012.

INTRODUCTION AND ACKNOWLEDGMENTS.

Cancer has probably plagued humanity more than any other illness down the centuries, and it was probably referred to as the Palsy or the Wasting Disease of the past. Today it continues to be complex, widespread and devastating. However, there are many positive rays of hope for the present and the future.

Research has led to new and much more effective treatments. It has led to more accurate diagnosis, and the development of amazing equipment. Continuing treatment for patients, and monitoring of peoples health, means that a recurrence of the disease is more likely to be detected. There is much more knowledge available about the prevention of cancer, and there are complementary therapies, and diet and exercise programmes to help patients.

It must be recognised and remembered at the outset that cancer can produce a number of different outcomes for patients. Tragically it will often result in death, though this event may be considerably delayed now due to new treatments. Some patients will live with continuing cancer, held in check by medication. Some will experience "remission" with the disease apparently having gone away. Some patients will be declared cured, though I do know from my own experience that this is not always the end of the matter.

It is hoped that this small book will be a practical help to all cancer patients. With such a vast subject, always facing changes, this book must of necessity omit a great deal. We hope it may also act as a "signpost" book, pointing patients to other sources of information, help and support, both in their local area and beyond. It must always be remembered also that tackling your cancer is a team effort, but you are number one in that team, for it is your body which needs care and healing at this time. This book will also particularly seek to help carers, on whom such a large burden always falls, and it will also talk about treatment and nursing care. We sincerely hope that it will make your present and future more positive as you combat the disease of cancer.

Without the help of others this book could never have been written, and we especially wish to acknowledge our debt to them. The inspiration for the book came from Louise Smith, Cancer Nurse Specialist, and manager of our Ipswich Cancer Information Centre. She has been an enormous help in preparing this book. We also sincerely thank Dr Jonathan Knight, Stacey-Anne Penny and her District Nursing Colleagues, Pauline Douglas and Friederike Englund from Macmillan Cancer Support, and Sue Hughes from Marie Curie.

Debbie Taylor, Senior Oncology Dietician, has helped us greatly, and we are grateful to Stephanie Alban and other cancer patients for their support and contributions.

Without our computer team to tame the animal, we should have sunk without trace! We marvel at the skills of Max and Clare Slater-Robins, Harry Robinson and Phil Tyler. Theirs is the talent, the mistakes are all our own!

Finally, once again, grateful thanks to our seasoned proof reader!

Tom and 'Tricia Tyler.

Ipswich U.K. 2012.

CHAPTER 1. BEING DIAGNOSED WITH CANCER.

As noted in the Introduction, there are very many different types of cancer, perhaps about two hundred in all. Further, these will range from the mild to the very aggressive, and there are few parts of the human body which cannot be affected either directly or indirectly.

Most cancer patients (though by no means all) will want to have further information about the disease which is now affecting them. They will want to know the nature of the cancer, and where it is believed to be located, and how much of their body is involved. They may at this stage also want to know about treatments, the likelihood of cure, and changes which may be required to their way of life.

Our amazing bodies are made up of cells, millions of them, and it is the function of these cells which can go wrong, meaning that they no longer behave in a regulated fashion. A cell, or small group of cells can begin to multiply and grow abnormally, and these are called a tumour. They will no longer perform the function they were intended for, and they can obstruct the essential working of the body. Such cells can also move to other parts of the body using the blood stream, or the lymphatic system, and cause "secondary" cancers. There are also haematological cancers, which do not form a solid tumour.

It is usually an essential preliminary to treatment, that the original or "primary" cancer is discovered, and this may sometimes be hard, as it was the first time I had cancer.

Many people will first suspect that something may be wrong with them because of a symptom which they notice. It may be a sore place that does not heal, or a mole on the skin that grows or changes shape. For a woman it may be a lump in her breast, or unexpected bleeding. A persistent cough or soreness of the throat can be a clue. Unexplained tiredness, loss of appetite or loss of weight can point to something wrong. When our bodies are in trouble, sometimes they will signal the fact by producing pain. In my own case the first time it felt as though a red hot poker was being pressed into the back of my neck. I had never experienced such pain, and it took strong morphine painkillers to bring me any relief.

Once diagnosed, most cancers will fit into a particular category, such as Lymphoma, Melanoma, or else they are labelled according to the part of the body which they affect, such as Ovarian, Breast or Prostate cancers. Cancers which affect the blood are usually grouped together under the title of Leukaemia. Other cancers will affect the bones, and need a special type of treatment.

While many of those who are diagnosed with cancer will want to find out more, as will their families and friends, this attitude will not apply to everybody, and there will be patients who decide that they do not want to be given any further details at all. They feel that all they want to do is place themselves in the hands of doctors and nurses, and simply "let them get on with what they think is necessary." Some of these patients may feel they do want to know a little more once their treatment is under way, and they have got over the trauma of the first diagnosis.

For some such patients, this handbook will be quite superfluous, and their attitude should be totally respected, even if those family and friends who are near to them honestly believe that the patient would be able to cope better with their treatment if they knew better what was happening to them and why. It must always be a matter for individual choice, and the choice each patient makes must be respected by family and medical team alike.

Whilst cancer is most common in those aged sixty five or over, it can affect a person of any age, including small children, where the illness will pose extra challenges for nursing staff and for the patient's family. Cancers will often be quicker growing and more aggressive when they affect younger people, but the positive aspect is that such cancers will often respond more effectively to treatment..

When someone is diagnosed with cancer today, they will find that the doctors and nursing staff will do everything they can to explain the exact situation with regard to the disease, as far as they know it, and to answer questions. Because of the pressure of clinical work, there must always be some time constraints, however.

To help fill any gaps, there are a number of other experts on the disease who can help, and give more time, such as specialist cancer nurses in Information Centres, radiographers or other allied health professionals and members of the Macmillan phone line teams. In addition Macmillan in particular have produced a comprehensive range of booklets which give a huge amount of helpful information. Patients should look for an Information Centre in the hospital which they attend, and make full use of its resources if they wish to. The Macmillan booklets are all free, as are many of the other services that are offered.

On a note of caution, patients should be slightly wary of the great Internet! The Internet is only as reliable and accurate as the people who post information on it. Sadly, because Cancer is such a widespread disease in its many forms, and because of its potentially emotive and devastating nature, there may be "remedies" peddled on the Internet which will not really help patients, and could even harm them if mixed with other medication. The only help given is to empty patients wallets for the benefit of the person who promises so much and delivers nothing. If 42% of our countries population will experience cancer during their life time, then cancer must be about the biggest business in the entire nation.

This first part of our handbook is written very much from a patients point of view, - in fact only this morning I have heard that my recent course of chemotherapy seems to have been successful, and I am in the clear. This latest experience of cancer and its treatment has been a sort of refresher course for me, following a much more severe experience about seven years ago, so I am writing with things fresh in my mind.

Because of the great variety of cancers already mentioned, diagnosis has always been a considerable challenge for doctors and consultants. Many cancers might not really produce distinctive symptoms, and could be confused with diseases such as tuberculosis in the early stages. By the time the true nature of the illness was discovered, it was too late for treatment. In days gone by, say forty or fifty years ago, the only thing a surgeon could do was to carry out an "Exploratory operation." In the case of one such patient, known to me, testicular cancer was discovered, and successfully dealt with, and he went on to have six more children and died many years later from a totally different cause.

But it must be said that all too often the surgeon would operate, take a careful look and then stitch the patient up again, sadly declaring that nothing more could be done. Often after such an operation had been performed, the decrease in pressure brought about would make the patient feel better for a time, before the disease took hold again.

Today we are amazingly fortunate, as there are several means of diagnosis which do not involve invasive surgery, other than perhaps a biopsy, and methods are improving almost month by month. It should be noted, however, that our cancer survival rates in the U.K. are at present considerably worse than those in many other European countries, and that early diagnosis is the key to improving these results. People should be "on watch" and at the first sign of any symptoms should attend their G.P. as soon as possible in case a problem is developing. The first type of medical tests for a patient are linked to blood analysis. Most test samples will be taken in your local doctor's surgery, or at the local hospital when you attend for an appointment. In the surgery you will usually be "sampled" by a practice nurse, and in the hospital you will meet a phlebotomist who is specially trained to do this work. Few of us actually enjoy having a blood sample taken, but the staff are brilliant at doing it, and I just offer an arm and look resolutely out of the window!

Analysis of your blood sample will be done at the hospital, and with the wonderful modern machines they have it takes hardly any time at all. The results will tell your doctor or consultant a great deal about the nature and extent of any disease which may be affecting you.

Perhaps the greatest advances have been made in the development of scanning machines, which have been greatly improved from the X-Ray machines of the past. We now have CT, PET and MRI scanners. The two former machines work using X-Rays, while the MRI scanner uses a magnetic field. Thanks to these wonderful machines the experts can build up a picture of the whole human body, including what is going on inside. The machine can focus on the area of a patients body which is affected with disease, and by the introduction of special fluids into the body, specific organs can be highlighted, and enable the machine to give an even clearer picture. I have just had a PET scan for the first time, and the results have been most helpful, - and hopeful.

The scanning machines will usually be found either in a hospital building or in a large mobile trailer adjacent to a hospital. Patients will be sent full details of their appointment and of necessary preparations, and also usually a map showing the location of the scanner. Preparation can require a period of fasting, 6 hours with the PET scan for example, and also drinking a lot of liquid.

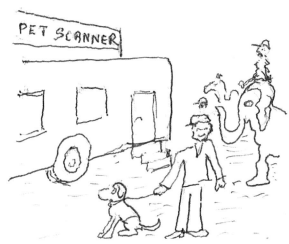

A PET scan does not require a pet!

The scanner staff are always most helpful and reassuring, and the procedure is really very easy. There are a few things a patient should know in advance, First, you may have to change your garments and substitute a hospital gown. If you are very fashion conscious this may present a challenge! Discreet changing rooms will be provided for the operation. Second, it is not always easy to get comfortable on the sliding "tray" which takes you in and out of the machine. Cushions and other supports will be available, however. You will usually lie on your back, and enter the scanner head first.

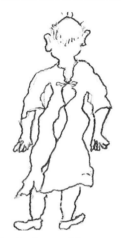

My fashionable gown!

Third, with some scans, notably CT and PET scans, some special fluid may be passed into your body using a "line" and cannula, or by injection. None of us like having this done, but it is an essential part of the scanning procedure. With the PET scan radioactive glucose is administered, but I did not notice myself glowing at all.

Finally, while the CT and PET scanners are shaped like a giant horseshoe, through which you pass, the MRI scanner is a tube into which the patient slides, and this may be a worry to those who suffer from a degree of claustrophobia, as many of us do. In addition, the MRI scanner, which will take about 45 minutes, is remarkably noisy. The staff will be most understanding and supportive if you tell them of your concerns and problem, and they can administer a mild sedative to help you cope with the experience of the scan.

With my recent PET scan the excellent staff made me so comfortable that I actually dropped off to sleep at one point!

While the experience of having one of these scans may not be a pleasant one, we must always remember that the benefits to us, the patients, given by these wonderful, - and highly expensive machines, are tremendous, and may well make all the difference to the type of treatment we receive, and its eventual outcome. It is well worth putting up with a short period of discomfort to gain such a huge benefit. There are excellent leaflets giving more detailed information about the various procedures, so do ask for one if you want more information.

After a scan has been done, there will be a period of waiting for the results, and this is a very worrying time, for one knows how much of ones future may depend on what the scan has shown. The result will usually be communicated by a doctor in the hospital, at a prearranged appointment. If the result of the scan shows a cancer, and as in my last experience this is a complete bolt out of the blue, it will leave the patient in a state of shock. This is why it is important to have someone with you for this occasion.

After the diagnosis you will return home, and there may be a delay while further tests are carried out, before the prescribed treatment begins. Meanwhile most patients feel that their world has been turned upside down, and they wonder what to do next. Who should they tell, and how much information is it best to give? What commitments in the diary should be cancelled at once, and which can be kept for the time being, until things seem clearer? What about work commitments, who should be contacted, and can work be continued, perhaps part time? You still feel exactly the same as you did yesterday, but is it wise to go out and mow the lawn which so badly needs attention?

Each of these scenarios will have its own set of complications, and every case will be different. Every household will be unique, and just as patients vary in age, so the partner and extended family will differ in age and outlook. For example, the decision to carry on at work, perhaps with reduced hours, will depend on your age, the nature of the work you do, and how you are feeling. Employers are very good usually when it comes to supporting employees diagnosed with cancer, and there are many healthcare professionals and others who can advise and even accompany a patient to talk to their employer. There is specific Employment legislation which protects the rights of a cancer patient with regard to their work. Details of such help are given later in this book. If an employee is suddenly diagnosed with cancer this will often be unknown territory for the employer, and there is the smooth running of the company to be considered, and the livelihood of other employees.

Again, with regard to domestic situations, there can be endless variations. In cases where there is a family, and indeed others, the patient and those around him or her may wish life to just go on as usual as far as possible, with as few changes to routine or household geography as possible. This can be a way of keeping the illness firmly in perspective, or even trying to pretend it does not really exist. It can underline a firm determination not to be beaten. If children are present it can be reassuring to them that all is well in their family.

Later I shall be looking at the problems of resting and sleeping while undergoing treatment, and suggesting some minor alterations in furniture, perhaps. Living as we do in a bungalow, such changes for day or night use have been easy to make, but I accept that for those in 2 or 3 story houses such changes may not be so easy. Each family will want to sit down and discuss the matter, and it is perhaps best not to do anything in haste. I would recommend that you meet each changing situation as it develops.

With regard to your attitude to your home and beyond there will again be significant differences. The first time I was ill I was really very ill a lot of the time, and my home represented my "security." I tended to hibernate there, knowing there was always a chair, or a bed, or a loo when I needed one! But this last time round I have weathered the treatment much better, and felt much more confident about going away, even having a couple of nights in a hotel on one occasion. However, the suggestion of a day on the beach did not really appeal, as I felt I should need to position my beach chair up on the promenade outside the gents conveniences!

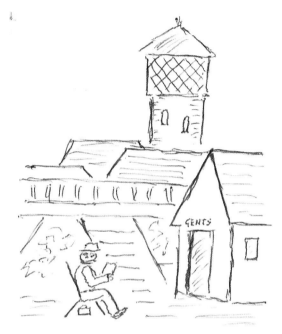

"Sitting outside the Gentleman's convenience."

Having said that, I know many cancer patients have organised holidays during or just after treatment, and greatly benefitted from the feeling of a return to normality as well as a change of scenery. Travel Insurance companies are usually very understanding, and holidays can often be postponed because of the onset of the illness.

Incidentally, while a patient may not want to go away from their home very much, it is wonderful when family and friends "pop in." Such visits not only bring a breath of fresh air, but reassure a patient that they have not been forgotten by the outside world. However, I have found in the past that the treatment has affected my voice, and I can no longer talk the hind leg off a donkey, so visitors should be encouraged to keep their visits to a reasonable time, and the carer present should watch out for signs of the patient getting tired, like dropping off to sleep in mid sentence! Most people will quite understand if someone drops a hint that the patient needs to have a rest period.

In a family where the patient is working, and the chief breadwinner, without pension income, there will at once be potential financial worries to add to the concern over the cancer and its treatment. In such situations there is a lot of help and advice that can be given, and for example Macmillan operate a Benefits clinic in our own hospital, as well as paying visits to patients in their homes. They have also given an enormous amount of help to benefit claimants, many of whom were unaware of what was due to them because of their illness. Macmillan will also make grants direct to cancer patients, preferably for specific projects, where appropriate. It does no harm to ask for help and advice. There is a section later in this book devoted to the work of Macmillan with cancer patients.

While the treatment of your cancer is inevitably going to have a significant effect on your usual life routine, there is no reason why it should completely take over, except in cases of extreme illness. In fact, as we shall try and show, there can be positive aspects to what is certainly a potentially challenging experience for every patient. However, it is terribly important to remember that everyone's journey through cancer treatment is going to be different, and what I have experienced on two occasions will be very different to your experience. Having said that, and I will try always to remember it, I hope that this book may yet be a help to you.

CHAPTER 2. THE LOCAL HOSPITAL.

There are two usual routes to becoming a cancer patient. The first is through your G.P. and your local surgery. You will make an appointment to see the doctor because you feel something is wrong with your body. This may be something very specific, like a swollen throat making eating difficult, or a more vague awareness of pain or discomfort.

It should be remembered that despite a large caseload, the average G.P. will only come across a handful of definite cancer cases in his surgery each year. Cancer may be a widespread disease, but there are many other illnesses which may give similar symptoms. However, if you as the patient suspect something is really wrong, you should persist in asking until you have an answer which gives you full confidence. If the G.P. decides to refer you to a consultant at the hospital, you should receive an appointment within two weeks, and if you don't do so, ring up to find out what is happening.

The second route to becoming a patient is through a routine screening process. Such screening has been available for breast check ups for a number of years, but new techniques are being developed to detect other cancers in the early stages, including the use of specially trained sniffer dogs. If a test shows cause for concern, you may be directly referred to the relevant consultant at your local hospital.

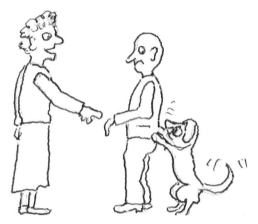

You're not getting cancer – she can smell
the kipper in your pocket

In the event of a rare cancer, the patient may be sent to a specialised hospital further away, perhaps even in London. For most potential patients their first port of call is the local hospital which has a department which will specialise in their particular problem. In my own case first time round it was an orthopaedic surgeon, but there will be head, neck and throat consultants, as well as specialists for breast, prostate, ovarian and gynaecological, liver and lung cancers. Those with suspected leukaemia illness will find a special department for haematological cancers, where they will be treated using the appropriate treatment. Skin cancers will usually be treated in the dermatology department.

As a patient you will be attached to one department and looked after by its staff, who you will get to know well. But it is always helpful to remember the many other patients being looked after elsewhere, and whichever department you are in, it is a good idea to seek out the Cancer Information Centre in your hospital, if one is available, or contact the local Macmillan telephone support line.

Even when provided with a map it is quite daunting to find your way round your hospital, unless you already know it well, but there will be reception desks where you can ask the way, and some hospitals have volunteers waiting to greet you and give you directions.

As well as having a consultant and doctors, each cancer patient should be allocated to a specialist nurse. This nurse will be a specialist in your particular type of cancer, and will act as a link between you and the consultant and the team. If you have a question or a problem this is the person who should be contacted first.

Once tests and scans have been completed, the patient will have a meeting with the consultant or a registrar doctor, and will be told the type of treatment being recommended by the hospital team, where the treatment should be carried out, and who will supervise it. Do make sure someone accompanies you to such a meeting to take notes for you, as there may be a lot of material to assimilate.

It is usual after such appointments for a further visit to be arranged, and this can be done at the reception desk, although you will also receive a letter of confirmation from the hospital in due course. The hospital may provide you with a folder containing a lot of most helpful information, but it is also advisable to have a file to keep letters and other papers in, and also to have a diary which you keep up to date and refer to every day. There may be a lot of appointments to record over the coming months and there are many of us who feel that chemotherapy and other treatments do not improve our brain power, and our ability to forget has never been better!

It is to be hoped that your local hospital is not located too far away from your home, as when you are feeling unwell travelling is not a lot of fun. Further, the cost of running a car, and of parking at hospitals can be considerable as the weeks go by. Do make enquiries either at the Oncology Department reception desk or the Cancer Information centre about help with hospital parking charges. It is a good idea to make a note of the direct line telephone number for the centre, and remember no question is ever too trivial. I should also mention the Macmillan Cancer Support phone line, which is staffed by cancer nurses, and a great source of help and support.

During this period when you are having your first appointments, and then beginning treatment, either the Oncology department, or another department, will inevitably become a focal point in your life and routine. In regard to this people tend to divide into two groups.

First, there are those who find all aspects of hospital procedures and treatments threatening and uncomfortable, and even at times very painful. With regard to pain, it should be stressed that we all have differing "thresholds of pain" over which we have little control. However, much can be done, and will be done by hospital staff to help those who find treatments painful. But for this first group it is utterly understandable that they can dread their visits to the hospital, however skilled and kind the hospital staff prove themselves to be.

The second group of patients find that they can put themselves into the hands of the doctors and nurses, and just let them get on with whatever has to be done. It does not necessarily mean that their experience of treatment is any easier or more comfortable, but it does bring a sort of peace of mind to just "go with the flow." The hospital staff are very good at explaining what is being done and why, subject to the usual time constraints, but again there will be a significant number of patients who really do not want to know, and their wishes will always be respected.

If the cancer patient is considered to require treatment involving chemotherapy, hormone, radiotherapy or nuclear medicine, then this will be given in the Oncology department, which has a staff trained in every aspect of cancer treatment, and where further tests may be done, treatment planned, and the treatment given to the patient.

The Oncology department in your hospital will usually have its own reception desk, where you should report that you are present, and a waiting area. From here outpatients will be called in turn, and shown to a consulting room or a treatment room, depending on what the patient needs.

Also in this department there will be a hospital ward for inpatients. If you are to become an inpatient, you will be notified in advance, and night things etc should be brought. The ward is often used by patients having their first treatment of chemotherapy, so that they can be kept in for observation for a night, and it is also used for more seriously ill cancer patients.

The radiotherapy unit will be part of the department, perhaps with a separate reception desk, and waiting area. Modern radiotherapy machines are very accurate and sophisticated, and the very skilled staff will explain to each patient what is happening and what they are required to do. The same thing applies to the nuclear medicine department. Incidentally becoming radioactive for a short period is not painful, and the effect wears off very quickly.

After using the facilities in the oncology department the patient will very soon find their way about, and the staff will become personal friends. I certainly now regard this part of my local hospital as a home from home, and I am extremely glad it is just down the road from where I live. It gives me a great sense of security!

While the hospital will of necessity play a large part in your life at this time, it is also most important to maintain the link with your G.P. and to keep him/her informed of your progress. I have found that an occasional phone call is much appreciated.

CHAPTER 3. METHODS OF TREATMENT.

This is a chapter which some cancer patients may feel they do not want to read, and if that is the case do not feel you have to!

Following the tests and scans the oncology team will then discuss the results and decide which treatment will be best for each individual patient. There are six main forms of treatment.

A. SURGERY. Depending on the nature of a patient's tumour or lump, and especially where it is located, surgery may be the ideal option. The patient will be admitted as an in-patient to a surgical ward at the hospital. You will have the suggested procedure carefully explained to you, and be asked to sign a consent form. You will be visited by the doctor who will administer the anaesthetic for the operation. Then, following an injection, you will go to sleep and know nothing about the operation until you wake up in the recovery room, feeling a bit sore and possibly woozy in the head.

The length of your stay in the hospital will depend on the seriousness of the operation, and the amount of aftercare that is needed. It is policy today to get patients out of bed and walking about as soon as possible, to help recovery and avoid possible complications. During this period monitor how you feel, and do not be afraid to report any pains or problems to the staff. They can do a great deal to control pain, and help your recovery in other ways. Remember that some of the pain killers you may be given will produce almost instant constipation, so watch out! Again, the staff can help you with this problem.

B. CHEMOTHERAPY. This treatment involves a cocktail of drugs which can be administered to the patient in tablet form, by injection or by a drip. The "recipe" for each patient will be worked out by the consultant, aided by other experts, and the dose is usually mixed up shortly before it is to be administered.

Most treatments of chemo are given in the outpatients department by a drip. You will be seated in a comfortable armchair, with your arm supported on a pillow, and a nurse will insert a cannula into your arm through which the fluid will pass. The nurses are brilliant at doing this, and you will hardly feel it happening. The fluid used is contained in a bag

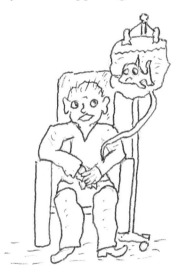

which hangs from a pole on wheels, and it passes by gravity into a machine which carefully regulates the flow, and keeps a score of how you are getting on. The bags of fluid may be changed at times. The procedure doers not hurt at all, and it is a good idea to bring in a paper or good book. Drinks will be provided, - it is important as always to drink, but you will need to bring in your own food, snacks, sandwiches etc.

When we are finished Nurse, I will have that fish with some chips!

You can get up and move about if you have to, and you can walk your bag trolley to the loo when necessary. The treatment may take anything up to several hours to complete, - my record was about 12 hours on one memorable occasion, and then it is a good idea to have someone else to drive you home, as you can feel a bit wobbly! I shall talk about side effects in the next chapter.

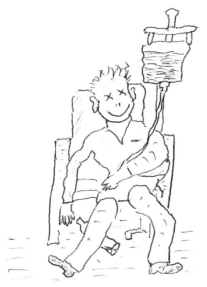

Nurse, will you check what Mr Blotto has got in that bag.

Each chemo treatment is called a cycle, and the consultant will tell you how many cycles are planned for you. These are given at regular intervals, say every three weeks. A scan may be done at half time, to see how you are getting on.

C. RADIOTHERAPY. This form of treatment uses high energy rays to eliminate cancer cells, and it may be used as a "back up" after chemotherapy or surgery, to be sure that your cancer has been removed.

First, the patient will be asked to attend the radiotherapy department for "marking up." The staff will explain what is happening, and will then examine your scan results and mark on your body with a coloured dye exactly where they want to point the rays. They will then make an appointment for your first treatment, and these will usually take place daily. They can be interrupted if you have a commitment that cannot be changed.

For the treatment you will lie on a type of bed, and the radiographer will arrange your position as required. The staff will then retire to a cubicle, and the machine will move into position, and when everything has been checked the treatment will be given. This is painless, and only takes a short time. When it is finished you will be able to go straight home. Again, side effects will be discussed in the next chapter.

D. HORMONE TREATMENT. Your body manufactures hormones, and these are important for it's development. Unfortunately they can also aid cancer cells to grow. This form of treatment, usually administered in tablet form, at home or at the hospital, aims to combat the misuse of hormones by the cancer cells. It is particularly used for prostate cancer treatment. Again, the treatment will be given in cycles, and the side effects discussed later. The staff will monitor the effect of the treatment and decide how much should be given.

E. BONE MARROW TRANSPLANT. Your bone marrow is a most important part of your body, and it contains all that is needed to make healthy new cells. Bone marrow can be damaged by chemotherapy, and by other disease, and the result can be the cause of leukaemia or other blood disorders. To correct this situation an operation called a bone marrow transplant can be performed. This will be done in the hospital, where you will be an inpatient, and the same sort of procedures as for surgery will happen. Much progress has been made in recent years with this type of treatment. Again there are excellent booklets which give more detailed information if you want it.

F. BIOLOGICAL THERAPY. This is sometimes referred to as "Immunotherapy" as the method uses the body's own natural defence system to fight the cancer, with the help of biological products. It is a relatively new way of combating the disease, and clinical trials are still taking place. Administration of the drugs may be done by injection or in tablet form, and the procedure will not be painful. Patients will be treated usually as outpatients, but the effects of the treatment will be carefully monitored by the hospital staff.

Other powerful drugs like steroids may be given in addition to chemotherapy treatment, and will need to be taken for several days at home. These can also affect a patient's body in various ways. They can cause nausea, acute thirst, weight gain, and even trigger diabetes in some people, though this is often temporary.

CHAPTER 4. SIDE EFFECTS OF TREATMENT.

If you have a normal cycle of chemotherapy treatment you will spend part of one day at the hospital outpatients department, and twenty days at home feeling the after effects of the treatment. The other forms of treatment detailed will also affect your body in different ways.

   When I was given my first treatment of chemo, the drugs affected my heart quite badly, and I was told by a heart specialist "if you have more chemotherapy, you will die from a heart attack." Fortunately for me my two brilliant oncologists refused to be beaten, and by experimenting with the chemo recipe discovered which drug was the culprit. So here I am! Heart problems are comparatively rare as a side effect of treatment, and as shown they can be sorted.

   Side effects could be divided into two closely intertwined categories. Physical, such as taste, appetite, nausea, hair and weight loss; and mental, such as anxiety and stress, and fatigue. Some of these subjects will be dealt with in subsequent chapters, as they are most important for a patient.

  It must again be stressed that we are all different, and the same treatment will affect different patients in different ways. In fact some people will hardly encounter side effects at all, while others can feel really ill.

  Many people will feel nausea after treatment, and particular drugs can be taken to prevent this feeling. This can also be linked to a loss of appetite, and a change in taste. Some things which have always been your favourite foods suddenly taste pretty horrible. Those like me who have been very fond of their food can go right off it, with consequent weight loss. The disease and treatment can leave you looking gaunt and grey, and very obviously a cancer patient. This happened to me the first time round, but not at all the second!

We shall look at diet in a further chapter. Another result of chemotherapy can be whole or partial hair loss. For those of us going bald, it is no great matter, for women it is a very big factor in their feeling of wellbeing, and there is lots of help and advice available for them. In our Cancer Information Centre there is a section devoted to "Hats and Headgear" and this includes wigs. Special arrangements can be made with a suitable shop to provide wigs paid for by the NHS. It is important to remember that after chemo has ended the hair will grow back, and sometimes end up more healthy and prolific than it was to start with!

There will be other lesser side effects of your treatment. You can have a tendency to develop a sore mouth, and a special mouth wash should be used at least twice a day to combat this. Incidentally, I have found that chemo seems to be the cure for my mouth ulcers! After radiotherapy you can find a burning of your skin, almost like sunburn. A cream can help soothe this effect. In my case the treatment on my neck caused me to lose my voice for several weeks, - the family said it was a blissful period!

Hormone treatment can affect the balance of hormones in your body. It is usually men who have this treatment, and it can affect their voices, and produce a tendency to develop "breasts" which can be disturbing for some. Again, once the treatment is over things will return to normal.

In place of loss of appetite may come a considerable thirstiness, and drinking is always important during treatment, as it flushes out the kidneys. After one treatment I measured myself drinking a gallon in 24 hours, but I know that is pathetic by some beer drinkers standards!

Patients should be aware that sometimes dizziness can be a side effect, and be particularly careful when standing up quickly. It is good to have someone on hand when getting in and out of a bath, and using a shower with a stool or seat might be preferable. Patients should assess carefully their ability to drive a car safely, and have a word with their GP if they are worried.

The drugs used in chemotherapy, and the powerful rays used in radiotherapy can damage the nerve ends for certain patients. This can result in a condition called Peripheral Neuropathy. The symptoms are a sort of "pins and needles" in the finger tips and toes, and a feeling of deadness in the soles of the feet. Walking can actually become quite painful in bad cases, and don't I know it! You will also have a strong tendency to drop things, which doesn't help when trying to assist in the kitchen!

I believe some Complementary Therapies may help, but ultimately if the nerves have been badly damaged there is no cure for the condition. Complementary Therapies will be discussed in the next chapter.

One of the most important things when you are having treatment is to rest when your body tells you it wants to. Again fatigue and sleep will be discussed in detail later, as they are very important subjects.

To summarise, remember always that during these treatments, and especially chemotherapy, your body is taking a real bashing, even though you may not always realise it. The chemo is cumulative in its effect, so the side effects will become stronger and more pronounced as time elapses. You must "listen" to what your body is telling you. Eat when and what you want to. Rest when you feel tired. Adopt whatever daily routine seems to suit you best. Don't be afraid to say "no" if you don't feel up to doing something or going somewhere, - unless it is up to the hospital for your treatment. Some things are still compulsory!

Remember also that we are all different, and one patient's experiences may be very different to another's. Don't be put off by what other people tell you, even if it's in print like this! Never shrink from asking questions or reporting problems, as there are many many people out there only too ready to help you. Again more details later in this book, and remembers to write down on the blank pages useful names of contacts and their phone numbers.

CHAPTER 5. HOSPITAL APPOINTMENTS AND THERAPIES.

Hospital appointments may be made on the telephone or by email, but they will usually also be confirmed by letter. Do make sure you put the date and time in your diary. When you first attend at the hospital you will probably be given a loose leaf folder containing a lot of useful information. This will have been specially assembled to contain information about your particular form of cancer, as well as general information about the hospital and the oncology wing.

Do leave plenty of time before the appointment, and if you are travelling by car remember that parking at many hospitals is not easy and takes time, as well as pound coins!

It is most helpful to add a couple of blank sheets, and on these to record every visit you make to the hospital, and any important results or decisions that occur. Dates of chemotherapy treatments, scans, radiotherapy treatments and the like should all be recorded. You should also make a list of all medication that you are taking, and keep this in the folder as well. If, like me, you are uncertain how to spell some of the drugs and pills, do ask a nurse or doctor to write down the name for you. This can avoid certain confusion when you are asked, as you will be, about what medication you are currently taking!

When you are going to see a consultant or registrar doctor you may be required to uncover portions of your body for inspection. It is helpful if you do not wear a wet suit, or even many layers of tight fitting clothes! The doctor is not really interested in spending many minutes watching you struggling in and out of your clothing!

Do remember that the consultants and their staff see dozens of patients every day, all of them just as important as you are. They will give you as much of their time as you need and they can spare. But also be considerate over others who are waiting, and do not indulge in chat about the weather or your pets etc!

Once again a reminder that the specialist nurse allocated to your care should be the first port of call if you have any questions or something is bothering you. The local Cancer Information Centre and the Macmillan Support line are valuable sources of help also.

During and after your treatment you may suffer stress, discomfort and perhaps pain. In addition to the medication which you can be given, the hospital may be able to refer you for a variety of therapies to help you. There are also therapists who you can access privately, but do enquire about the cost first, and also discuss the idea with your doctor. Sadly some therapists are not as knowledgeable as they like to make out. I suffered from one such who was convinced my pain was the result of a sporting injury, when in fact it was a large cancer lump on my spine!

Most hospitals will have a team of physiotherapists based in the building, to whom you can be referred. However, they are usually very busy with a large caseload, including many orthopaedic patients, and appointments may be delayed and limited. There are private physiotherapists available in most areas, but do make sure you go to someone who is experienced and properly qualified. Some therapists may not feel able to work on cancer patients, due to lack of training and experience. Physiotherapy can be a great help in toning up muscles which have been affected by treatment for cancer, and also when a patient has been unable to take much exercise due to fatigue.

Some hospitals will also have a team of complementary therapists who work part time at the hospital. You will need to make appointments to see them, and this is usually done at the reception desk. The therapies which are offered may include:

ACCUPUNCTURE. This is an ancient therapy, coming from China originally, I think, and involves piercing the body in certain places with small needles. It sounds uncomfortable but I am assured this is not so, and many people maintain that it has very beneficial results. There are practitioners in some hospitals.

MASSAGE. This can be applied to the whole body or parts, including the head, hands and feet. It is especially good for the relief of muscular aches and pain, and will induce a feeling of wellbeing. A masseur will usually use special oils, suited to each patient, which have their own healing properties. The masseur will also have a special table, and be able to make the patient completely comfortable. Again, many hospitals have masseurs working within the hospital framework.

REFLEXOLOGY. This therapy works on the belief that our feet are especially connected to other parts of the body, and that a special type of foot massage will benefit the whole body. Having experienced it a number of times I can testify that it certainly works for me! For this massage the patient will lie on their back, suitably supported, with the feet bare.

REIKE. For this therapy the practitioner will pass his or her hands over certain parts of the patient's body, but not actually touch the body. The therapy relies on the belief that energy can be transmitted to parts of the body that need it, and patients testify to the help this gives them.

ZERO BALANCING. This seems to be quite a new therapy, and like some others the therapist will manipulate the patients arms and legs, soothing muscular pain. A special table is used.

RELAXATION THERAPY. Here the therapist may read or recite a story, which has a strong visual and peaceful content, while patients are encouraged to relax their muscles and breathe more deeply. It is recognised that stress and anxiety affect our bodies and wellbeing, and that a therapy which thus reduces stress is most beneficial.

VISUALISATION THERAPY AND COUNSELLING. In this case patients are encouraged to visualise situations and problems which are troubling them, and to write about them or talk to a counsellor about them. Doing this often reduces the level of stress and worry.

There are many other therapies, which may be beneficial to some people, but patients should always check the professional credentials of therapists, and if possible always seek the recommendation of either a doctor or the hospital. Having said that, I have personally been greatly helped by some of these complementary therapies.

CHAPTER 6. AN INPATIENT IN HOSPITAL.

It may well be the case that during your treatment for cancer, of whatever kind, you will spend a few nights as an inpatient in the hospital. For those who are "old hands" this is no big deal. But for many it will be a new experience, and a few tips may help.

Remember that being a patient in hospital is a partnership between you, the patient, and the staff. Many hospital wards these days are understaffed, and anything that patients can do to help themselves is much appreciated. Lying in bed and constantly ringing your "nurse summons" bell will not make you at all popular. But if you are specifically told to stay in bed there is a reason, and you will not be commended if caught straying down the corridor.

Most hospital wards work to a fairly strict routine from Monday to Friday. Early to mid morning, consultants and doctors will do their very important rounds checking on all patients. Ward matrons will want their wards clean and tidy, and this applies to patients too! Breakfast eaten, washing done, beds made, lockers tidy are part of the drill. Drugs will be given, and some other treatments. Visitors will not usually be admitted during this period.

Mention of lunch brings me to hospital food. In most hospitals catering is done from a central kitchen, and food taken to every ward in special heated trolleys. It is a big operation, and does not allow for a lot of individual choice. Food is seldom like mother makes it at home! However, it is essential that as a patient you eat properly in hospital, and dieticians work hard to make sure hospital food contains what you need. Those of us trained at boarding school and in the army, long ago, can find the food extremely tasty!

Afternoon and evening on the ward are times for another meal, usually a light one, and two periods of visiting. Having visitors is the highpoint of the hospital day, but if you are not feeling well it can be very tiring. Most visitors realise this, but don't be afraid to drop a broad hint! Shutting your eyes and snoring gently usually does the trick.

Socializing gently with other patients is a great help to everyone, you included. Some patients may be bored, some lonely and fearful, some even rather confused. Talking to someone, or perhaps playing a game of cards with them or sharing a paper, magazine or book is a good way of helping, and with the usual wards of six beds it is easy to get to know your fellow patients.

In 2004 when I had several spells in hospital my top half was in considerable trouble, but my legs were OK and I was determined to try and keep those muscles fit. The staff were very helpful and kind, and I was allowed to walk the long corridors before breakfast. I paced the length, and tried to do two miles each day. The porters and cleaners who were up and at work thought I was quite potty!

Every inpatient lives for the day of escape! One weekend I felt well, so on the Friday tried to persuade my consultant to let me go home for the weekend on the grounds that my dog was pining for me. He looked at me for several seconds, then said "Mr Tyler, I have seen many a patient looking far better than you do, and they have been dead in twenty four hours."

I stayed in hospital, and it was a reminder that you are there for your own good, not to benefit the hospital.

CHAPTER 7. THE CANCER PATIENT AT HOME.

During and after treatment the cancer patient is likely to spend the greater part of their time at home, - probably about 99%. Home situations will vary greatly, as will family and friends, as cancer as we know is no respecter of persons.

Whoever you are, and wherever you live, as a patient you will have basic needs which become very important when you are a patient. You will need somewhere to sleep and to rest; somewhere to cook and to eat; somewhere to pursue hobbies and interests; somewhere to wash and visit the loo. We shall consider these basic needs in detail in later chapters.

Most patients will have to make the best of their existing accommodation, and in fact the presence of what is familiar and comfortable is very reassuring when you do not feel well.

Patients households will of course vary greatly, and the accommodation with them. Where there is a family unit, with dependant children, the needs of all members of the family have to be considered, and in fact the patient would want it to be so, therefore try to avoid any change which imposes strain and tension on the other family members. Children need to know what is happening, and why, but their lives need to go on as usual, with schooling and homework, sporting and artistic commitments taking place as normal.

The cancer patient may or may not be able to continue to drive, so it is to be hoped that their partner will be able to do shopping trips, and drive the children about. If this is not the case, it can present quite a challenge, especially over a period of months. If a patient is uncertain about driving, as I was, they should raise the matter with their GP. Most patients realise their limitations, and may feel they can manage local trips safely, but would rather not confront a motorway.

Because cancer patients are more likely to be in the 50+ age group, their children may have left home, and have commitments of their own. Most families, however, are wonderfully supportive towards a parent who develops cancer. Patients will divide into those who are living with a partner, and those who are on their own.

Those with a partner are fortunate as they have home based support, and even a degree of nursing care, - or in my case superb nursing, being married to a nurse. Being a cancer patient one is very aware of the support of others, even if the medication makes one feel unwell and at times downright grumpy! More will be said about this in the "Carers Section" but one thing is most important, and that is that carers/partners get a good night's sleep, even if the patient is up at frequent intervals or cannot sleep. Separate beds may be necessary, or even separate bedrooms!

Patients who live alone may hopefully be able to arrange for family or friends to be contactable on the phone, - mobile phones have made this more easy, and for others to do some shopping, mow a lawn etc. If friends can organise a rota to supply companionship that is a great help, though you should let sleeping patients lie! Remember too that patients on their own will have continuing needs even though their treatment is over.

There are many sources of support for patients in their homes, and later we shall point you towards some of them, but it has to be said that there is no substitute for kind and caring neighbours.

CHAPTER 8. DIET AND TASTE.

A persons diet is always of great importance to their health, but it is even more important if you become a cancer patient. Both the disease itself, and the consequent treatment, will put great strain on your body, and eating the right foods is one way of giving your body the extra strength it needs to combat what is happening.

I have received great help from dieticians when I was ill, and their advice has been invaluable. It should be stressed that a good diet is important all the time, and not only if you develop cancer, and the ingredients should be roughly as follows, dividing your food into four main categories.

1. Foods that provide you with starch, and fibre. These will include cereals, bread, lentils, pasta, porridge, and potatoes. They should be included in some form in every meal of the

day, and for most of us this is so. To pass through our bodies they will need to be mixed with fluid, milk or water being the obvious choices. There is an increasingly large choice for us now, and with the arrival of so many varieties of pasta as well it is not difficult to enjoy this part of your diet.

2. The second group are dairy products, including milk, butter, cheese, yoghurt, ice cream and so on. Custard is one of my lifelong favourites. Unfortunately I am told that milk chocolate does not count! These products provide us with fat, so should be included but rather sparingly. Many contain

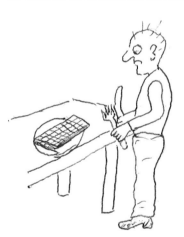

saturated fat, which is not good for the heart and arteries, but there are unsaturated alternatives based on margarine, and for those who have problems with dairy products there is a good substitute in Soya milk. We are actually incredibly fortunate with the range and availability of different foods today.

Unfortunately milk chocolate does not count.

3. Fruit and vegetables make up the third group, and here the message of "five a day" does seem to have registered. We are also advised that our selection should be as varied and colourful as possible. Again, it is not hard to include these in a daily diet given the wonderful range of fruit and vegetables

available, and you may even be fortunate and hard working enough to grow some in your own garden. My dietician says firmly that carrot and banana cake does not count as two of the five, and a glass of orange juice only counts as one, however much you drink! Again, variety is important, and being told that rhubarb may help prevent cancer doesn't mean you should eat nothing but rhubarb! That would probably kill you.

4. Finally there is the group of foods which give us our much needed protein, without which our bodies cannot renew healthy cells. This group will include eggs and nuts, fish, and white and red meat. For those who are vegetarian, substitutes will have to be found, and many are offered in our shops, such as beans, nuts, and pulses. Some foods like oily fish, mackerel, sardine and herring for example, have particularly good health properties. Advice is always being revised, and perhaps 2-3 portions of red meat a week is ideal. However, some people "down under" start the day with a huge breakfast steak! Also oysters may not always produce the desired results!

Much of your choice of diet is down to common sense, and old adages like "a little of what you fancy does you good"are probably perfectly valid today. Those who find that during cancer treatment they are losing weight, and for most of us this will be true, have permission to indulge in butter and cream, full fat dairy products, chocolate and biscuits, with a large slice of cake at intervals to break the monotony!

There are two factors which will contribute to loss of weight at this time. The first is a loss of appetite, due to the medication you receive, For me, always ready for my food at any time, it was utterly surprising to find I just didn't want it, and was pushing my food round the plate in a disheartened manner. This is the effect of the drugs, which as we know are very powerful. The second is the distortion of taste, which is caused by some chemotherapy drugs. Again it comes as a nasty surprise when the usually beloved cup of tea suddenly tastes like something passed by a Billie goat!

If you are lucky enough to have someone who prepares your meals for you, it can be very dispiriting for them to find you are losing weight and refusing the food presented to you, over which they have laboured long. They must be reassured that this development is no reflection on their cooking.

With regard to eating meals the recipe should be "little and often." It is important to have some breakfast, as this is the time when your body needs "fuel" to begin tackling the day, and it may often be the time when you take most of your medication. A bowl of cereal, with milk, will be a good start, and with the range of cereals available you should find several which taste good.

You should try and follow this with a snack mid-morning, some lunch, afternoon tea, and an evening meal. Some people will be helped to sleep by a small snack at bedtime, with warm milk, Horlicks etc. Some of this may be "comfort eating" but there is no harm in that. Eat what you fancy, and if something does not taste nice find a substitute. Using snack meals rather than elaborate main meals may also help.

If you are eating a sensible and varied diet, you should not require any special supplements, or vitamins, however heartbreaking that news may be for the food supplements industry. However, if you are worried talk to a local dietician, as there are good products which they can recommend for you, which will be in harmony with your treatment drugs, and won't cost you an arm and a leg.

With regard to alcohol, a patient will tend to get advice from different quarters, some of it conflicting. This last time I suddenly got a craving for a drop of cider with my evening meal. I asked my consultant whether a little cider with my chemo was alright, and he replied that it was fine as long as I didn't start falling over! The generally accepted belief is that a small amount of alcohol each day could be beneficial if you feel like it, but emphasis on the "small."

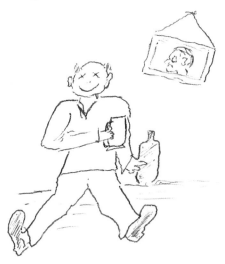

"Fine, as long as you don't start falling over!"

Your diet is going to be very important at this time, but do not get hot and bothered about it. Mostly it is a matter of common sense, and you should be eating a good balanced diet of food all the time if you value your health. Do not be phased by headlines that the most recent research suggests this or that food is the answer to cancer. The so called research is usually based on an absurdly small sample of people taken over an absurdly short time, and will be contradicted by a new piece of research reported on next week!

Finally, remember again that the great internet is only as good as the people who post stuff on it, and some of them may have a strong desire to sell you this or that!

CHAPTER 9. EXERCISE.

Just as a good diet is most important for your body, so is exercise. As I mentioned, I tried when an inpatient to at least keep my legs working. However, when being treated as an outpatient you will have lots of scope and opportunity to take exercise, and it is important to do this.

There are two methods of exercise, which are perhaps best mixed together. Formal exercise will involve attending a gym or swimming pool, or joining a cycling group perhaps, and exercising with a group, or with a trainer.

The type of exercise you take will obviously depend on your age, and also the treatment you have had – those who have had surgery will need to be very careful at first. For such, advice from a physiotherapist at the hospital should be taken, and exercise started very gently.

Gym training is very much in fashion at present, but not all fitness instructors are trained in helping cancer patients, so again care should be taken. At our hospital contact has been made with a number of fitness trainers who are anxious to help, and their qualifications have been approved by our professional staff. However patients should be aware that many gyms are only too anxious to recruit new members in order to improve their finances.

We have been fortunate to find a hotel sports and leisure centre who are happy to allow a group of cancer patients to use their swimming pool at a weekday time for half price. It is a quiet time, and during school term we almost have the pool to ourselves, and this is a huge bonus when some of our members may be self conscious about how they look. This not only enables patients to work on their physical fitness, but gives then renewed confidence and an ideal time to socialise with others.

We also have a cycling group coming into being, where the bikes are provided for members to use.

Informal exercise may take many forms, but chair exercises, walking, home gym exercises like a rowing machine or treadmill, jogging, or individual swimming are all possible and most helpful. Having quite a large dog ensures that I go out once or twice a day, and one can attempt "power walking" to raise the heart rate. Not everyone is lucky to have lots of local footpaths and beautiful scenery.

While it may not be necessary to have an actual exercise plan, it is important to try and make definite progress, gently stretching your physical abilities week by week, walking a little further each time, or swimming a few more lengths of the pool.

Recent research suggests that regular and manageable exercise will help a cancer patient cope with treatment, overcome symptoms sooner and help prevent recurrence. It is also suggested that when feeling fatigued it is not always the answer to retire to bed, - sometimes some gentle exercise will chase the fatigue away and make you feel a lot better.

In our "Moving on" group, about which more later, we are visited each month by a fitness instructor who suggests armchair exercises ideal for older patients and those who are feeling rather fragile. Again one must remember that those who are over 60s will feel the effect of their age after cancer treatment, and also conditions like Peripheral Neuropathy may affect patients, - my feet are sometimes so sore that walking is not easy. Luckily the dog is happy to walk quite slowly as well!

CHAPTER 10. FATIGUE AND SLEEP.

These two related subjects are of great importance to all cancer patients. Many patients suffering from a range of medical conditions will say "I can cope as long as I get a decent nights sleep." Unfortunately both the disease, and the treatments used to combat it, will usually affect sleep patterns and produce fatigue for cancer patients.

Fatigue is not just an increase in tiredness, it is a long term feeling of exhaustion, which recedes and develops with no relation to what the patient is doing. It is hard to be specific about the cause, but for most of us it is the effect of the disease, the effect of its symptoms, and the effect of the powerful drugs used to treat the illness. It may be a combination of all three, and usually is.

Most patients will find fatigue affects them in similar ways. You will find that at times you feel quite normal, and can tackle a new day with reasonable energy and enthusiasm, if not with gusto. You will be tackling the chores, and suddenly feel the need to sit or lie down, and take a breather. Once resting, you feel that you will not get up again. The thought of spending the rest of the day in bed is most attractive.

This fatigue can not only make your body feel without energy, but in some way it will sap the energy in your mind, making you lethargic, unable to concentrate, and even forgetful. Most cancer patients feel that the illness or its treatment have a definite effect on the mind, and I have found that my ability to add up a column of figures isn't what it used to be. I hope it comes back, or I shall have to invest in a dreaded calculator!

Those who are supervising your treatment, or administering it, should warn you about the likelihood of fatigue. The first and most important rule is "do not fight it." If you feel fatigue, you must leave whatever you are doing and go and rest. Second, if you feel it necessary, speak to your GP or the staff at the hospital, and ask their advice.

During my recent spell of chemotherapy treatment I kept a chart of my fatigue and sleep patterns. I noticed that both were in step with the particular phase of my cycle of treatment. I also noted quite clearly that the feeling of fatigue was cumulative and after five treatments I felt far more fatigue than after a couple.

With respect to fatigue, the patient should not take to their bed for the duration, as this will tend to cause other problems. The answer lies in a combination of determination and low cunning!

When you are feeling tired or perhaps a bit depressed, a great deal of time and mental energy can be spent trying to remember what you intended to do next! The answer is that simple but much derided device, the List! Either in bed with a cup of tea for stimulation, or at the breakfast table, draw to yourself a folded A4 sheet, head a column with the day and date (things easy to forget, - if you are a bad case you can add your own name as well to jog your memory!) and then list the things you would like to get done in a column, with gaps for elevenses, lunch, tea and supper. I always end my list with "bed" which I find very reassuring.

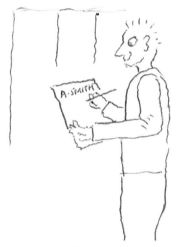

"Add your own name as well to jog your memory!"

The next step in your cunning plan is to arrange the tasks to be done so that you have a mixture of things which will require some degree of physical exertion, interspersed with tasks that can be done at the kitchen table or in your comfortable chair. And again the golden rule applies, in addition to a period in the early afternoon designated for "rest" you must also take a break if you suddenly feel tired.

Again, the way you cope with fatigue will depend a lot on your home situation, If you live alone, or live with a partner, or have dependant children, your situations are going to be very different.

If you are alone, some chores like hanging out washing, shopping, gardening and cleaning the house can be especially onerous. Do not be reluctant to accept help that is offered or even solicit help where necessary. If you can afford to have a cleaner for a couple of hours each week, spoil yourself! This may apply especially to men on their own?

Cooking for those on their own, and feeling very tired, and also for carers who may feel very weary may be made easier with some tips. Don't feel you have to provide elaborate feasts at frequent intervals. If your partner has lost his/her appetite they won't be appreciated anyway. Little and often, with simple meals is a much better strategy.

Make full use of the microwave and the freezer if you have them. When cooking a macaroni cheese or mince, cook a larger size portion, and freeze half of it for another meal in a few days. But remember to label things in the freezer or you can end up with mince and custard by mistake!

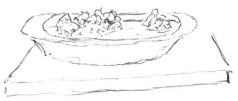

"Mince and custard by mistake."

I have to admit that when I am on my own I use the minimum of cutlery and crockery, and the dishwasher does make washing and drying a lot easier. Also standing at either the cooker or sink can be tiring. It is better to sit at the kitchen table when preparing food, and picking apples and blackberries can also be a testing experience!

If you have dependant children, and they are of an age to understand the situation, talk to them and enlist their help. Most children will rise to the occasion once they understand the problem and are asked to help. Sometimes their eagerness to help can be quite overwhelming, and very touching.

If your children are younger, then you will need help with childcare. Use a pram or buggy to help transport, not only for children but for their equipment as well. If outside employ the wheelbarrow! While one cannot just employ anybody, do accept reliable help over childcare, taking children to and from school and to playgroups. When combating fatigue, it has to be a case of taking each day at a time. It is also important when making your list to have some sort of priority system, perhaps marking with a cross items which need to be done first, and leaving others to be done tomorrow if need be.

One important aim of the list and priority system is to try and reduce stress and anxiety, and enable a patient to be as relaxed as possible.

As already stated, gentle exercise can often reduce fatigue, but even so there will be many occasions when a cancer patient needs to rest. This can be done on a bed, perhaps with some favourite music, or sitting up watching the bedroom television – if you have one, or reading a book. In such a situation it is easy to shut the eyes and have forty winks. Try and have a phone handy, or disconnect it, and determine to ignore the front door bell.

I find it most useful to have another relaxation location, and this was greatly assisted when my wife decided we should buy a recliner chair. Here I can have a book to hand, and also watch television, old video films, of which we have hundreds! – favourite music, a jigsaw puzzle on the go, and a pack of playing cards. In addition I have a wonderful view out of a large window, and with a pair of binoculars can watch the wildlife in my garden. This year a hummingbird hawk moth and a golden eagle have been the high spots!

The result of this strategy is that even when resting you have the feeling of doing something positive. Resting in bed or chair is not a sign of defeat, but more a positive use of time for entertainment or education. As you go to bed, you can look back on a day well spent.

If you are able to continue at work during your cancer treatment, albeit perhaps on a part time basis, you will also need to have a strategy worked out. This must be discussed with your employer, but most will be very understanding and supportive. There will be two main features here. The first is to do your work in short periods, with time to rest every now and then. Obviously some work is much easier to do than other types when you are feeling fatigue. Being a blacksmith, or a professional tennis player will present special challenges!

The second tactical priority is to create a quiet comfortable place where you can rest. This may be a room set aside for staff, or even a storeroom. If such a place does not exist on the premises it may have to be your car in the car park. Try and park in a secluded place, and have cushions and a blanket to hand. In winter you will need the car heater on at intervals. You may be able to listen to the car radio or read a book for half an hour. A thermos of tea or coffee is always welcome. As with so many things, planning ahead is the key.

A very high percentage of cancer patients face sleep problems, which will increase as the treatment progresses. As with fatigue, I also kept a sleep pattern chart during my recent course of chemotherapy treatment, and again it was quite interesting.

I had my chemotherapy treatment at 3 week intervals, and was able to receive it without interruption this time, unlike my first experience. On the first night after the treatment I did not sleep at all. Going to bed at the usual time, I tossed and turned for two or three hours, then got up and retired to my recliner chair. I am sure that this was the effect of the drugs that had been administered, and especially perhaps the steroids.

In my case, during recent treatment, the usual pattern of sleep was restored after a couple of nights, but I can still wake up at 3.a.m. and lie awake for a couple of frustrating hours, as I did this morning. For many recovering cancer patients the problem is much longer lasting, and can result in long term tiredness, and even despair. Taking sleeping tablets on a regular basis can make one feel like a zombie the following day, so is not a permanent solution.

Although we are all different, there are some ideas which may be a help. Try to keep to a routine, going to bed and getting up at the same time, and aiming for seven to eight hours sleep a day. Time your meal times so that there is a three hour gap between eating your last full meal and going to bed. Avoid late night tea, coffee or other stimulants. (This may be a challenge if you are invited out to supper!)

Try to take a reasonable amount of exercise every day, and if you feel the need of a nap in the middle of the day, make it after lunch, and for a limited period, - set an alarm clock! At night try to ensure that your bedroom is an even pleasant temperature, - you may need to use a fan on hot summer nights, and try to keep noise levels to a minimum, - not easy if you live next to a main road!

It goes without saying that a truly comfortable bed is essential, - after all you may be going to spend one third of the rest of your life there! Zip and link beds mean that the hardness of the mattress may be different for each partner, and also if you move about in the night your neighbour is less likely to be disturbed.

Finally, there is Plan B. If you are going through a period when your sleep pattern seems shot to pieces, and you dread going to bed at night, this may be a help. In your lounge/living room set up your most comfortable chair, preferably a recliner type, facing the television. Have a duvet or blanket handy depending on the time of year, also a glass of water, favourite book , even a jigsaw puzzle. Have several well loved music CDs or DVDs ready to put on, and some old films on video or DVD.

When you go to bed you no longer have to peer at your bed with a feeling of anxiety, - what will the night hours have in store for me this time? You can think of all the treats waiting for you in the other room, and almost wish you will wake up at 3.a.m. and be justified in getting at them! However, the chances are that you will get a good night's sleep.

If you do find yourself awake with no prospect of sleep, you can creep out of bed, taking care not to disturb a partner, put on a few clothes, migrate to the Plan B location, chose what entertainment you fancy, and then make yourself warm and comfortable in your chair and get ready to enjoy what remains of the night hours. It may well happen that in half an hour you are sound asleep with Mozart still playing gently, but it doesn't matter if you are not, as you will have made positive use of the time. In the morning you can take your partner a cup of early morning tea with a virtuous feeling, and the knowledge that you have had a rather "special" night, and watched an old film you enjoyed very much indeed.

For most of us this problem with our sleep pattern is a temporary thing, and as we recover after the treatment has ended, the problem will certainly recede, if not entirely go away. For some patients, however, the problem will persist, and they should seek professional help. Again, as with other things, do make sure the person you consult is truly qualified, and not a D.I.Y. "expert" whose main ability is charging outrageous amounts of money per session.

Much research is being done on this problem of sleeplessness, so do not give up if it is your problem, however much it is getting you down. Your local Cancer Information Centre, or local Macmillan nurse will be the best places to ask for advice.

CHAPTER 11. RELATIONSHIPS.

Relationships with those around us, near and far, are always somewhat complex. If we accept the premise that the basis for a relationship is some kind or degree of love, then we might accept the definition of C.S.Lewis in his book "The Four Loves" where he divides love into four kinds, Affection, Friendship, Eros and Charity.

When a patient is diagnosed with cancer, the news will ripple outwards among all those with whom the patient has a relationship. Because until quite recently, as we have already recalled, a diagnosis of cancer was almost considered as a death sentence, those with a relationship linking them to the patient often did not know how to react to the dreaded news.

Should they cut off all communication, on the grounds that "any mention of such a horror was abhorrent?" Should they write a letter of deep condolence, followed up with flowers via Interflora? Should they think of another excuse to write, but make no mention of the medical news at all? Or should they write acknowledging how shattered they also feel, and offer any help they can? Or, if living close by, should they bake a large cake, take it round, and share in a huge hug and a lot of tears?

A lot will of course depend on the strength of the relationship, which is why Lewis makes the sub-division between affection and friendship. Affection is that feeling experienced by people who are acquaintances, perhaps business colleague, or sporting companions. People you meet regularly in the shops or at meetings. They are people who will be so sorry to hear the news of your cancer, and will want to know in due course how you are getting on. Some of these, through the experience of sharing your ordeal, may well become friends.

Friendship implies a bond of love. Friends are people who stand by you, who weep with you when you weep, and rejoice with you when you are joyful. Even so, some friends, and family, sadly, will find the news of your cancer very hard to deal with. I often hear stories from cancer patients who have found that when they told a friend or family member of their diagnosis, there was a total and immediate break in all communications. We usually say, a little glibly perhaps, that "It is probably because the person just does not know what to say" and is taking refuge in silence. But I do sometimes wonder. If a person is a true friend, whether family or not, how can the bond of love which exists just be cut off? And especially when the person who has just learnt that they have cancer is in need of all the love they can get?

For someone who has just become a cancer patient will be acutely aware of the friends, near and far, who are upholding them in love. Telephone, text, letters, quick visits, whether with a cake or not, offers of help, doing shopping or being a private taxi, weeding in the garden, - there are so many ways a patient may experience the love of true friends, and I have been so helped myself by experiencing this..

The relationship of friendship is not just a warm glowing feeling when you are with someone, a recognition that someone is a special chum. It is actually a very demanding relationship to be a friend, and it will involve pain, and truth, and sacrifice, and even sometimes rejection. But heaven help those who face cancer, - or many other things, and who have no friends. We should never take friendship for granted, for of all things it is one of the most precious.

We now come to Eros, the intimate love of two people, and this will spill over into the next chapter as well. Many cancer patients will have a partner or spouse, and sometimes this relationship will have been a long one stretching over many years with many differing experiences. In addition, there may be close family, children, parents, grandchildren. The central unit of two partners will be closely affected by these closest members of the family.

Two main and powerful ideas will have to be taken on board. First, not only will the disease have its effect, but as has been stressed, so will the treatment. To single out three things, tiredness, irritability and depression often set in as a result of treatment. The patient cannot help being affected by these things, however much they may resist, - and it will be those who are closest who tend to get it "in the neck!" The patient's partner is already under strain, perhaps more so than the patient, and these factors will put great strain on the strongest and most tender relationship.

Secondly, the arrival of cancer can be a sort of bereavement, especially if it develops later on in life. If a couple are, say, over fifty, they will already be finding that there are things they can no longer do, or wish to do, though hopefully there will be compensations in other directions. The arrival of cancer accelerates that process of thought, making them fear that the patient may not see children or grandchildren grow up, that they will not be able to cope with travelling, challenging holidays, keeping the garden tamed and so on.

Powerful thoughts such as these will be uppermost in the minds of both partners, and will occur to other family members as well. Sometimes those in close relationships prefer not to talk about such subjects, and this can naturally produce tensions between partners. It is never easy to broach subjects like these, but it is much better if they can be discussed.

I have just been told, in the presence of my wife, that I have "A handful of years left, probably." I am not quite sure how many years go to a handful, but given the incredibly shortened period between one Christmas and the next these days, it won't be that long! I am grateful for a frank assessment, but now the best way is to make fairly light of it, and to live each day to the full. When you think about it we all have a handful of years left, by and large.

If you are fortunate enough to have family and friends when cancer is diagnosed, you are indeed fortunate, and as far as you can manage it, as a cancer patient, appreciate this treasure and be thankful for it.

This is where we move on to the final one of the four loves, Charity. This could be defined as loving someone with no expectation of a love returned. Of truly wishing every good and blessing for someone, and doing what you can to bring your wishes for that person to fruition. This is perhaps the greatest and hardest of all the loves, and cancer patients and their carers can always look around them and find someone who is even worse off than they are.

If you find that your relationships are under exceptional strain, do seek help, either by talking to a close and trusted friend, or to a professional counsellor. It never helps to bottle things up, especially when as a cancer patient you have many other concerns and challenges to cope with.

CHAPTER 12. SEXUALITY.

Remembering "No sex please, we're British" this may be the chapter you decide to skip, or it may be the first you turn to! I realise that for some this chapter will not really be relevant, while for others it will be most important. Here again cancer can bring about a sort of bereavement, - a loss of a sex life that has been part of the patients self since puberty, and at times a particularly important part.

When those recovering after treatment for cancer are asked about what goals they hope to achieve, many will say "I want to put the clock back, to return to a normal lifestyle." This will include a return to a normal sex life, though this will seldom be mentioned, for we British are a little coy!

Two factors have to be taken into account. First, the treatment used to fight cancer, as already stated, has quite a devastating effect on the body, and the powerful drugs used with their legacy of nausea and fatigue play havoc with our sexual drive and feelings. Most patients will be quite resigned to this during treatment, and hope for better times later. However, there will often be a partner to be considered, and it is most important that their feelings and needs are taken into consideration.

With regard to the physical side of cancer treatment, help can be given to both women and men by health care professionals, but remember not all health care professionals are trained to help in such situations, and many may feel embarrassed to offer advice.

The cancer drugs can cause physical problems which interfere with sexual intercourse, such as dryness of the vagina and erectile dysfunction. Both these situations can be helped a great deal, and in my case a small yellow pill prescribed by a doctor at the hospital was excellent. The only problem was that it was suggested I take half a pill, and I found that when bisecting them in the early morning with my scalpel, both halves were inclined to shoot sideways at speed. Trying to extract half a pill from under the cooker before the dog gets hold of it is rather a passion killer!

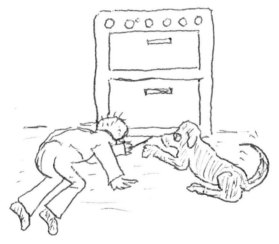

"Competing with the dog."

For cancer patients who are younger there can be every expectation that you will resume a "normal" sex life once your treatment has ended, and your body has had time to settle down again, but do remember that this can take some months, and don't be worried if things take time to return to normal. Do explain to your partner how you feel, and talk things over, and if necessary seek the help of someone like the most expert therapist who works in the sexual health department of our hospital.

The second factor that has to be born in mind, if you contract cancer when you are older, say over 60, is that if treatment and its aftermath takes a year or two, you will be that much older at the end of it, quite apart from the effect the disease has had on your body. You cannot reasonably expect to put the clock back exactly.

In our younger days we are stimulated by exciting films, magazines perhaps, rather graphic books even, and thoughts can turn to nights of passion, sexual gymnastics and remarkable (and physically impossible) positions, even to creating "artistic" films of our acrobatic performances. As the years pass our attitudes can change. Now the big "C" stands for Comfort. Your foreplay can better be eight hours of peaceful and untroubled sleep, followed by a lovely morning cup of tea, while your after play will be another hour of sleep while you recuperate and regain enough strength to get out of bed!

For most older couples a sense of proportion and a sense of humour will come to their aid, and their sexual relationship will be just as much fun as it ever was, and at times more so!

Again, all couples where one is a patient recovering from cancer can find help if they need it, and there are good books which will suggest simple ideas and be very encouraging.

It does need to be borne in mind that a number of cancer patients, especially women who have had breast cancer, may have had painful surgery, and be suffering continued pain or discomfort for many months as a result. The prospect of a male partner, who has become several tads heavier over the passing years, bouncing up and down on top of her is likely to be a definite passion killer, if not actually very painful. In my case the cancer left damage to several vertebrae as well as a disabled hand and arm, which is not a help where comfortable positions in bed are concerned. As a rule, like others I have talked to, I can only lie in comfort on one side.

Again there will be professional people who can advise, or books that can help. There are definitely some positions for intercourse which will not be helpful, and each couple can have fun experimenting to find what is most comfortable, - the big "C" again! One very suitable position for older couples is for the lady to lie on her back, with her head on a pillow. Her partner then lies on his side, facing her, and almost at a right angle, like the top of a "T." If the lady then raises the leg closest to her partner, bending her knee as necessary, they will fit together like two pieces of a jigsaw puzzle. I am an expert on jigsaw puzzles, so I know what pleasure they can give one!

Whatever the age of a cancer patient and their partner, the comfort which comes through intimacy, whether full sexual intercourse or embracing and caressing one another will be a great help in the battle against the disease. For those not in a relationship, meeting friends and family can also be a great help in fighting the feeling of isolation and depression which can threaten to overwhelm a patient. Loving and being loved are very strong and basic instincts for all human beings, and this is a time when such bonds and emotions really come into their own to help us.

CHAPTER 13. TWO UNMENTIONABLE "Bs."

This I have to say is a chapter I would much rather not have to write, but sadly I should be letting you down if I did not spill the beans, so to speak.

These two subjects, not mentioned very much if at all in polite society, and which can loom very large for cancer patients, are bladder and bowels. Whether we like it or not, and to be absolutely honest we do not like it, the effect of cancer, and of the subsequent medication or treatment used to combat it, can cause havoc with what was once a well regulated and organised internal economy. For some patients the necessary surgery to cure their cancer may produce extra pain and discomfort in their lower regions.

Those who have chemotherapy treatment, accompanied by steroid drugs, for example, can suddenly become very thirsty indeed. This last time round I decided to do a test and measured every drop I drank during the first 24 hours after treatment. I found that I eagerly consumed just over a gallon of liquid. I thought that was a lot, until a huge beer drinker on the T.V. informed us that he downs 18 – 20 pints on a Friday night alone!

Because, when you are having treatment, it is good to flush out your system, drinking a gallon is considered a good achievement, yet the results of all that fluid travelling through can be quite uncomfortable and debilitating, and can torpedo a good night's sleep.

Some treatments can cause irritation of the bladder and a consequent loss of control at times. This is usually not too serious, but it can be a nuisance. A patient feels reluctant to be very far from a loo during the day. When invited to spend a day on the beach with the family during my recent treatment, I declined the invitation as I visualised myself sitting all day in my folding chair just outside the entrance to the gentleman's convenience on the upper promenade!

Small and very discreet incontinence pads for both men and women are easily obtainable, and restore a feeling of security. They can be worn by day or night. Ask a district nurse or Macmillan nurse for help if you need it, but again don't suffer in silence.

If you find it is painful when urinating, you may have an infection, and should go to see your doctor, or else consult your specialist nurse at the hospital. The problem can usually be quite easily solved with a course of antibiotics.

I feel I am making a major issue out of this problem, but I know I am not alone in having to carefully plan a trip out to the shops so that I know where I can make a pit stop if necessary, and it often is. But take heart, like so many other side effects, the problem is definitely getting better now that my treatment is a couple of months behind me, and as with so many other situations, a return of confidence helps a lot.

Now we have to move on to the bigger challenge, if you will pardon the expression, and that is bowels!

It was not for nothing that apothecaries in centuries past studied the stools of their patients, in order to help them with their diagnosis. All of us need a gentle and efficient intestinal function, and when that does not happen we quite soon know we are in trouble. Those patients afflicted with bowel cancer may have to endure surgery, which will be painful and disruptive. Fortunately through the skill of surgeons, and with modern drugs, this condition can usually be tackled successfully, and the patient can hope for a near return to normal working.

Where things come as more of a surprise is when your cancer is, say, located in your neck, as mine was, and you yet find yourself engaging in the battle of the bowels. This is usually because you will be taking pain killing drugs, both as part of your treatment, and to enable you to relax and sleep, and most of these drugs are based on Morphine, and Morphine has an almost immediate constipating effect. It must be pointed out that occasionally it goes the other way, and a patient is smitten with diarrhoea, which is just as unpleasant, if not more so.

I have found that there are two courses of action, depending obviously which condition you are fighting. In the case of diarrhoea, there are several very effective treatments, obtainable through the doctor or from a chemist. The skill lies in taking enough to clear up the problem, without tipping things too much the other way. It is probably better to take too little medication to start with, rather than too much.

Constipation can be fought with two weapons. The natural one includes fruit, and in particular the famous prune, together with plums and apples, and plenty of fibre in the diet, washed down with lots of water. Of the medicines on offer, I found Lactulose effective and quite gentle. The secret is that if you know you will have a problem in this direction, anticipate it before you start having treatment. Twenty four hours before treatment go onto a diet of "prunes in Lactulose" (not found in most recipe books, I am sorry to say!) and this may well contain or at least greatly alleviate the problem.

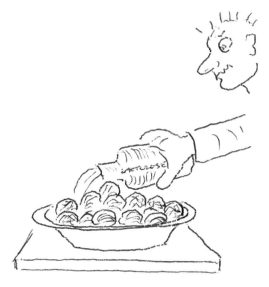

"Recipe for prunes in Lactulose."

Both these conditions can cause soreness around the rectum, and if you are a sufferer from the dreaded piles, then you may be susceptible to further troubles in this department. If that is not bad enough, chemotherapy can cause a weakening of vital muscles, leading to occasional incontinence. However, as stated before, it is not all bad news as the use of a small and very discreet pad can solve that one. Do seek help, and don't accept the need to sit two inches in the air above your chair, or perch on half a dozen cushions! If possible have a nurse or nursing trained friend who will help you combat your soreness.

The good news is that many of these problems are worst when you have just had your treatment, and things will improve after a few days, - until the next treatment. And the best news is that once treatment has finished, and the effects of the drugs have worn off, almost everything will get back to normal. If it doesn't, seek help!

I have found these problems some of the most difficult to cope with, especially when you have so many other challenges and worries, and are feeling decidedly unwell. While you are at home enduring your treatment, bladder and bowel situations seem to take over your whole life, by night and day. While as I have said, this is not considered a sociable topic for conversation at mealtimes, you will find family and friends are both understanding and very sympathetic, and you can sometimes make a joke of your predicament, and say that you are just training for the Olympics, or else trying to get into the Guinness Book of Records, - though in fairness I must warn you that I shall be a very hard man to beat!

CHAPTER 14. CREATIVE HOBBIES, SPORTING ACTIVITIES.

We have noted that the typical cancer patient will spend the majority of the treatment period at home, although there will be those who can continue at work, either full time or part time, while treatment takes place. There will be those also who work from home much of the time, and who will want to try and keep things going as far as possible. There will also be those who feel really ill for most of the time that they are receiving treatment, and who will just want to rest and do the minimum that is necessary to keep going.

I have already suggested that trying to have a positive outlook, and engage in some sort of exercise and creative hobbies, is a big help and for two reasons. Being positive, which is far from easy, does give us a feeling of uplift, of being on top however bad the treatment is making us feel. Also, finding creative hobbies of some sort helps to pass the time, as just sitting around doing nothing makes the long hours drag by.

As you may have gathered I am a great one for lists, especially when chemo or other treatments have robbed your brain of its full efficiency, - if it ever had any! Make a list of all the hobbies you have ever enjoyed dabbling in, and the sporting activities that you enjoy or have enjoyed in the past. Such lists can go back to making model aeroplanes or emulating Robin Hood as an archer! I would divide such a list into two parts, indoor and outdoor.

When you are having treatment for cancer, as I have indicated, you do tend to want to stay at home for much of the time, and this will be particularly so if it is the colder darker half of the year. Also, home gives you a sense of security, - never far from a bed, chair or loo! But there are so many things you can do at home which not only help to pass the time, but will give you a great sense of achievement, and may prove an introduction to something new you have never done before. I feel, also, that there has never been such an exciting choice of hobbies and pastimes, all easily available on the internet or through the post.

Because it is "sexist" these days to suggest that this is most suitable for women, and that is more appropriate for men, I shall mix all the ideas up! Actually, that is correct, for both sexes can have a go at anything given a bit of daring and enthusiasm!

Let us suggest you do not have a lot of energy, and want gentle things to do in your comfortable chair. With a lap tray you can play patience card games, read or write letters, - a "Kindle" will make reading easier, perhaps, if the latest gadgetry does not worry you. You will need a larger tray to do jigsaw puzzles, or if you are able to play games with others. Grandchildren are always ready to play board games given the opportunity, I find.

Other hobbies which can be very creative, and can be located in your favourite chair are embroidery and tapestry sewing, using perhaps the large range of kits available. Perhaps you can design your own picture to be worked, using graph paper? Knitting, sewing and lace making, - the latter very challenging but deeply rewarding, can be added to your repertoire. I have much enjoyed designing and sewing tapestry kneelers for local churches. Then we come to indoor hobbies which will demand a change of scenery. Today, it seems that every other T.V. programme involves cooking, or eating, or both. No wonder obesity is supposed to be becoming a huge problem throughout the nation!

For many, and especially those living alone, we recognise that just cooking for one can be an exhausting chore. So this is not for you! But there are so many new recipe possibilities, contained in books and on line, and not involving Jamie Oliver talents or resources! And after your experiment has turned out a huge success, friends and family will be delighted to help you eat the results!

Many of us have a conservatory, or small spare bedroom which could become a studio for the duration, and where pottery, painting, drawing, carving and sculpture can take place, as well as model making. It is a good idea to have adequate ventilation to reduce the smell of paint and glue! I painted my first picture for 18 years and much enjoyed it. Upholstery, toy making and making cards are all easier than you might think, as long as you begin with something easy.

You could try your hand at a patchwork bedspread, or set up a small aquarium so you can watch the fascinating behaviour of beautiful fish. There are coins or stamps to be collected, always an interesting hobby, and birds to watch and record in the garden. Then there is the realm of music, with old and new recordings, and a wonderful variety which you never normally have time to listen to. Make a list of things you would like to do each day when you are having your breakfast.

If you are fit enough during or after treatment, and you have the time and opportunity, there are outdoor activities, near and further away. Gardening is perhaps not for everyone, but on a sunny day it is wonderful therapy, and it doesn't matter if your garden consists of lawns and beds as far as the eye can see, or half a dozen pots on a small patio. Do as much or as little as you feel inclined, and the plants will reward you. Growing plants from seed is very fascinating, and not difficult to do, while even pruning can give you a lot of satisfaction.

Getting out and about a bit is good for morale and helps to pass the time and give a sense of achievement. For many the starting point may be walking a dog. Cycling is a wonderful way to get about, good for exercise, good for looking at the view, and saves a small fortune on motor fuel! But if you are a bit wobbly on the bicycle, then the car can take you to attractive places and give a change of scenery. We are so fortunate in our country to have a wealth of museums and stately homes within easy range, - unless you live on the Outer Hebrides, and there are places all over the country where outdoor activities like rowing and fishing can be tried.

Most of us are within reach of nature reserves, both for birds and mammals, or both, and which cater very well for those who have mobility problems. I always find I need to carry a couple of extra cushions. Some places provide excellent mobility scooters free of charge, which are great fun! In many parts of the country there are river trips available, and this is a wonderful way to see the countryside.

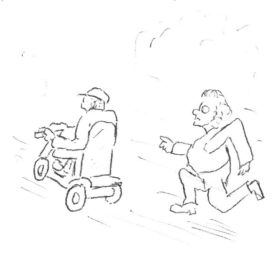

Excellent mobility scooters.!

In most areas there are clubs and societies that you can join, and where you will receive a warm welcome. These include wives groups, Probus clubs and pensioners clubs. You will probably find quiz nights and whist drives not too far away. In fact there is something out there for everyone, if you feel strong enough and so inclined. I have certainly found it a great help to get out and about a bit, though gently, during my last dose of chemotherapy treatment.

CHAPTER 15. OTHER SUPPORT FOR PATIENTS.

All cancer patients will need and appreciate support, as we have suggested. The amount and type of support will depend on two things. Is the patient living alone, or in a house with another person, or several others? Then second, how ill is the patient, both during treatment and immediately after it has finished?

Apart from the support and care given by the local hospital which is carrying out the patient's treatment, which we have detailed, what other support will the N.H.S. offer to a cancer patient?

The first place to look for support will be your local doctor's surgery. Although the doctor will have handed over your care to the hospital, as described, he or she will still be involved in your care, and especially in helping with problems which are a by product of the cancer treatment. But it is not always advisable for cancer patients to attend their local doctors' surgery, and especially if it is that period of the chemotherapy cycle when the patients blood count is affected, and they are vulnerable to picking up infections. This is the last thing a cancer patient needs to happen.

Not long ago the leader of a U.K. government gave great publicity to his "Care in the Community" initiative. It was the excuse to close down a lot of hospitals, and decant their patients back into their communities, where we were assured they would be cared for henceforth. But by whom?

In the past the local doctors could draw on the District Nursing service, and also arrange through these nurses for carers to visit those who needed help at home. The tragedy that I have witnessed is a running down of the nursing service, through lack of finance and lack of recruitment, and at the same time a reduction in the service which carers are allowed to offer. The latter are not even paid for their travelling time between visits, and sometimes in rural areas this can be a considerable part of the working day. I am sorry to suddenly become a bit political, but the result of this lack of "care in the community" means that a cancer patient cannot expect regular and frequent visits either from a Community nurse, or from very hard pressed carers.

Fortunately for many patients, relations, neighbours and kind friends help to bridge the gap. If the patient is a member of a club or church, they can expect to receive help, and others are only too happy to offer assistance. Don't be afraid to ask, as the grapevine does not always work, and people may easily be unaware of your situation. If people do not ask for help, others do not have an opportunity to give it, and it is exactly what you would do if the positions were reversed.

More will be said elsewhere about the work of Hospices, which have become such a blessing to our country over the years, and all as the result of the initiative and dedication of Cicely Saunders. At first they primarily offered care and support to those who were dying, but in more recent years this care has been extended to helping with palliative care needs, which is a very valuable source of expert help. A local

Hospice will often be able to run a day centre for cancer patients, who can be brought in to the centre once or twice a week. This has huge benefits for patients in giving them a change of scene, interaction with other patients, and a break for their carers.

Hospices will often offer respite care if they have accommodation available and most hospices which now offer Day Care in a Day Centre, through the "Hospice at Home" scheme will support patients in their homes. This is a highly valuable service, and you should be ready to explore it if you feel it would help you.

Macmillan Cancer support will be given more space elsewhere in this book, but here it should be mentioned that they give a great deal of support to cancer patients, including help with Benefits advice, and even grants of money to help with the costs of a holiday, for example. Macmillan advisers will visit a cancer patient at home, which is a huge bonus, and this also helps the advisor to better assess the patients circumstances, and possibly to notice other help that could be arranged.

The other group of specialist nurses who may be able to give support are Marie Curie nurses, who are paid for by donations and fund raising by the public. Their skill and expertise are of particular value to cancer patients who are facing a tough battle, but are still able to be at home. The Marie Curie service is limited, of necessity, and the nurses specialise in nursing cancer patients at night.

One area of support which some cancer patients may need is childcare. Children can be very helpful and supportive, as we have noted, but help with childcare, including trips to and from school, may be very valuable. It is best if this can be "delegated" to a close friend or relation, who will organise a rota of help, and supervise it. This takes the burden of worry off the cancer patient.

In the area where I live there is the ICAN support group for cancer patients, which meets in a church hall not far from the hospital. This group offers talks by visiting speakers, and outings and holidays, at very reasonable cost, and it provides a friendly environment where cancer patients can talk to one another, enquire about problems and progress, and give one another friendly support. The group is run by volunteers, but with a healthcare professional from the hospital usually attending it's meetings. Such groups are a wonderful resource, and can be a regular means of support especially to those who live alone.

In our hospital there are Myeloma Support and other groups, which are run by group members with the support of the particular specialist nurse, and we even have a Peripheral Neuropathy group, which sounds a bit mystifying, but is a great help. In another area I know of a group called "Bosom Pals" for those who have had breast cancer, and I am sure there are such groups across the country.

Again, in order to find out what is available where you live, you should contact your local Cancer Information Centre and they should have all the details to hand. Macmillan is also a very useful source of information, and will be able to give details of local groups.

The experience of cancer will confront a patient with consideration of their own mortality. Alternatively, it will make us consider the mortality of someone we love, someone who is very close to us. Whether you have some kind of religious belief, or none at all, it is hard to resist the temptation as you lie awake in those long night hours, to get out whatever belief you have, blow the dust off it, perhaps, and ask yourself whether it has anything relevant to say to you in your present situation.

There are many people who believe that death is the end of life for humans on this planet, and that there is nothing to follow. It is as if at the end a candle is blown out. Thus there is no need to worry about a future at all, and as you die there may just be a few regrets about things you would have liked to have achieved.

At the other end of the spectrum was Mrs Bruce, then aged 96, and living in a small room on the attic floor of a nursing home. I sat with her during the last hours of her life. All her family and friends had already died, and she was totally alone in the world.

"I'm so sorry you have no-one to be with you at this time" I said to her. She was quiet for some moments, thoughtful. Then a big smile lit up her face. "Just think of that wonderful crowd waiting to welcome me" she whispered.

Those who are believers, of whatever religion, will derive immense comfort and support from two sources. They will believe that God, in whatever form they recognise him or her, will give them whatever they need to endure and fight the ordeal they are presently confronted with in this life. They are not alone, for a greater power overshadows them. They will also take huge comfort and strength from the knowledge that friends and family, who are believers, are praying for them at this testing time.

All hospitals have a group of chaplains who minister to the needs of patients, and if your own religious faith is not one of the more usual ones, the chaplains will know where to seek the support and counsel which will be of most help to you. A message asking for a meeting can be sent via the ward staff. There will also be a hospital chapel, used by different denominations, where regular services are held for those who can attend them. Times of services will be advertised on the wards, and friends and family of the patient are always welcome to attend. In addition, chaplains will always come to visit patients on the hospital wards, and will conduct a service at a patient's bedside.

For those cancer patients at home, with a religious belief, remember that every house in Britain is geographically within a parish, and so has a Roman Catholic and an Anglican parish priest, and also can have a Free Church minister. Whoever is your local minister, he or she will do all they can to find the help and spiritual guidance which is most appropriate for you. I have to say that if you don't succeed at first, try again, more forcefully! There are also many helpful books, booklets and leaflets, so do please ask! You will have enough on your plate as you fight this illness, without tying yourself in spiritual knots worrying yourself about the exact nature of heaven, or whether they allow dogs there, (I am quite sure they do!)

I said to "The Major" who was dying of heart failure in a hospital bed, and seemed to want to talk, "Would you like me to say a prayer with you?" (I was dressed in clerical attire at the time so he knew who I was.) He thought for a few moments, looking rather uneasy.

"Well, Padre" he replied at length, "I really don't seem to have had much time for God in the past, and it doesn't seem cricket to go bothering him now, just because I'm in a spot of bother."

I know that on two occasions as a cancer patient I have been grateful for all the help I could get, and the future will be much the same, I guess. One must not let pride get in the way of asking for help from any and every source. It may come as a surprise, but the help, both human and divine, is there for the asking.

CHAPTER 16. REBUILDING YOUR LIFE AFTER CANCER.

One of the modern terms I have had to learn speaks of a cancer patients "Pathway." In this instance, I have to recognise, sadly, that the pathway has a fork in it, which means that for many cancer patients there will be no rebuilding of their lives in this earthly life. Therefore for many, tragically far too many, this chapter will not be directly relevant.

For most of us, when asked "what are your goals after cancer treatment?" the answer will be along the lines of "I want my life to get back to what it was before the disease affected me." This is a very good goal, as it can encompass mental activity, physical exercise and wellbeing, family relationships, creative hobbies and much else. But it may not always be realistic, - it hasn't been in my case.

Two important things have to be factored into the equation. The first is the possibility of continuing symptoms and consequent illness. Symptoms can include nerve damage, - the Peripheral Neuropathy already mentioned, which causes tingling and "pins and needles" and even pain in more severe cases. We have noted sleeplessness and fatigue, and also problems with appetite, and certain foods. The doses of steroids given during treatment can trigger Diabetes, as well as other complications, and chemotherapy can cause heart problems, in my own case ending up with a pacemaker.

It is impossible to produce a list of each and every ailment and symptom which may occur, and I do not want to present a pessimistic picture, for many people suffer very few if any after effects, and can feel after a few months that they are physically pretty well back to normal. In our swimming group for recovering cancer patients we have already seen remarkable progress not only in swimming ability but in general confidence as well.

The second matter to be remembered is more difficult to assess. If the cancer patient is in the under 40 age group, the body has remarkable healing powers, and strength will return once treatment is ended. Between say 40 and 60, though it is very hard to generalise over age, people may well find lasting physical effects of the disease, for example with regard to physical stamina and sexual libido. You will have to pause more often when digging the garden, and jogging will not have the same attraction.

For those in the 6o+ age group, things become hard to measure. Having had two bouts of cancer at age 64/65, and 71, I find it very hard to assess what has been the effect of the cancer on my body, and what is the effect of being seven years older. As none of us knows "what would have happened" it has to be a matter of conjecture, but one thing is certain: you can't put the ageing clock back, much as you would like to!

However, this does not mean that you cannot rebuild your life after cancer when you are 60+, the only thing will be that it may be a rather different building to the one that existed before the cancer. Having said that, it may be a much improved building!

For those patients with families, children and perhaps grandchildren, an important priority for the future is always given as watching family grow up, and being able to share in their achievements, as well as help with their problems. Having cancer makes one aware of the importance of family even more than before. For some, recovery means the renewed possibility of travel to see family, either at home or abroad. For those travelling abroad, whether to visit family or for a holiday, the question of travel insurance will come up. To get travel cover a lot will depend on where in the world you are headed for. Europe, Africa and the east are much easier than north America and the Caribbean.

Further, most insurance companies will not insure you for a "pre-existent medical condition" which means your cancer. However, because you have had cancer diagnosed, treated, and you continue to be regularly monitored, you are a much better insurance risk than many other people. There are a lot of people walking about in airport terminals who do not know they have dangerously high blood pressure! You should shop around for insurance, to get the cheapest quote, and don't worry about the pre-existent cancer, which is very unlikely to give you trouble on holiday out of the blue.

Most cancer patients, when fighting the illness and having treatment, do not feel like going on holidays. Now is the time to make up for that! Try something you have never done before, but which friends or family have enjoyed. Since we are now blest with the Channel Tunnel, it is possible to go by rail to a very large area of the world, though I am not quite ready for the trans-Siberian railway! Both coach trips, in very luxurious vehicles, and river cruises, are on the doorstep without needing to fly anywhere. Recently the wonderful variety and beauty of the British coast and countryside have been "rediscovered" by thousands of visitors. They are right here on our doorsteps, and the internet makes searching and booking very easy now.

Then there are the attractions on the very doorstep. The sound of birdsong on a spring morning, which makes waking up early a positive thing. (And don't be satisfied with a recording!) The changing seasons, acres of bluebells you never had time to stop and admire.

As you rebuild your life after cancer, do not forget to factor in time for relaxation and rest, with moments just for thinking. "What is this life, if, full of care, we have no time to stop and stare?" Having cancer is not the ideal way to tune up your priorities, but it does often have that effect.

There may be some things needed in your rebuilding programme which you would rather were not there. For many of us there are corners in the house where things lurk that should have been turned out years ago! Take heart, for even a trip to the local tip can be a very cathartic experience, at least so my wife tells me, and a car load disposed of at a car boot sale can actually be a lot of fun, apart from having to get up so early in the morning! You might even go a step further and consider redecorating in places, or even a much discussed alteration to the building.

Don't confine yourself to digging the garden, but do a bit of planning and improvement. As a result of my first cancer we tried chickens, than moved to a greenhouse and home grown vegetables. Now I am trying my hand at publishing books, and you may be able to assess the results for yourselves!

One result of having cancer the first time has been the opportunity to work as a volunteer in our local Cancer Information Centre, and this has been one of the most fulfilling things I have done in my entire life. I shall return to this subject in a later chapter.

CHAPTER 17. MOVING ON AFTER CANCER.

While a cancer patient will hopefully spend most of the time at home while having treatment, the local hospital will remain the source of support, advice and medical assistance. But eventually the moment may come when a consultant says "We have done all we can for you now. The last scan we did showed everything seemed to be clear, so off you go and we will see you again in three months."

The patient feels a great surge of relief, but when he gets to the door of the hospital this is replaced by a feeling of "HELP!"

Hospitals are now recognising that at this point in the cancer pathway, patients still need a lot of support, and as a result a national N.H.S. Survivorship Project has been initiated, with my own hospital as one of the ten pilot sites. This project required a lot of feedback from patients, in order to research the best way to help them, but in our case our local specialist nurse manager decided to go a step further and hold group meetings every week for recovering patients, in the local Cancer Information Centre.

We decided to call this the Moving On course, because we liked the idea of people moving on in their lives after the experience of cancer. Once you have had cancer you can never put the clock back, and the experience becomes part of your life history, and often a very large part.

But you must move on. You still probably have a lot of life to be lived, and as we have stressed in the last chapter there are lots of opportunities out there. The "Moving On" course we run is designed to help patients take the next step after treatment. They will meet weekly, for a four week programme, each session lasting two and a half hours. We have a half hour break for lunch, which we provide. This is a simple buffet lunch, and it is much appreciated. More important than delicious sandwiches is that it provides a "social period" when the group members talk to each other, because it is obvious to us that members help one another just as much as we help them.

We have specialist nurses and others who come to talk to the groups, and the topics covered are very much those we have already mentioned in this handbook, - diet and fitness, relationships and sexuality, stress and anxiety, continuing symptoms, travel and returning to work. The groups are an ideal opportunity for members to ask questions or share concerns. Our nurse specialist director of the programme provides the ultimate expert help, especially on medical matters, and also provides continuity between the groups.

At present, at the end of 2011, Health Care Specialists and cancer patients are being trained, where suitable, to be facilitators for a new programme, called the "HOPE" course, which is being sponsored by Macmillan Cancer Support. Again, patients who have finished treatment will be encouraged to share problems and look forward to a restored quality of life, wherever possible.

The Moving On programme has now spawned other groups which patients can join. We have forged links with a number of private gyms and fitness clubs in our area, and we regularly refer patients to fitness instructors who are experienced in helping recovering cancer patients, for either group or more often one to one fitness sessions. We are in process of organising a cycling group, again to help with fitness and confidence.

We have now established links with a local Care Farm, a member of the national network, and we hope that small groups may be able to visit the farm to find out whether this is beneficial to members. One of the farm staff is an ex-member of our Moving On programme, so there is an enthusiastic local link with the farm. We have also been helped by a local hotel which has a Sports and Leisure centre, and they are allowing a group of our ex-patients to go swimming every fortnight at a half price rate. This is going very well, and is much enjoyed by our members. Once again it is not just the swimming to help us get a little fitter, but the opportunity to meet and talk together which is proving so valuable.

One member of our group who was diagnosed with breast cancer, and then went on to have surgery, treatment and breast reconstruction, has kindly shared thoughts about body image and concerns.

1. It is difficult to look at oneself in a mirror naked, when one side of your body looks different to the other.
2. A woman will always worry that she is no longer attractive to a partner or boyfriend. We men should be aware of this, and do our best to help.

3. There is a strong desire to keep oneself covered up at all stages.
4. It is often difficult to find bras which fit correctly, and are comfortable to wear. (Don't be afraid to ask for advice from the experts, there is a lot of help available.)
5. You will tend to be continuously conscious of your appearance, especially at first. Can others guess you have had a mastectomy and reconstruction? Again, others, family and friends can do a lot to reassure you. You will be aware of what has been done for you, but it is highly unlikely that others you meet who are not in the know will notice anything at all out of the ordinary.
6. She admits that since her highly necessary treatment, she finds it difficult to be sympathetic towards those who have cosmetic surgery to enable their breasts to qualify for the Guinness Book of Records!

It should be mentioned that those who have had surgery for Bowel Cancer, and have to use a "Stoma" bag, may have similar and most understandable problems with body image. Again there are excellent specialist nurses to help patients cope with this challenge.

Our programme director is very keen that we should all have goals in life. We have already noted a good many of those in previous chapters, but for most patients "getting my life back to normal" usually sums up their goals. At a recent meeting of the "Moving On" group we had much the usual response, until we got to Tony, one of the older members of the group. When asked about his goals, he replied
"I want to master the geometrical theories of Apollonius." There was a slightly stunned silence, but luckily the name rang a faint bell for me, and I was able to link him to Euclid.

"My problem" continued Tony "is that there is only one book on Apollonius and his Geometry, and that has been long out of print, and I can't find a copy anywhere."

"Have you tried Amazon?" someone asked.

Tony looked rather bewildered, as though he couldn't believe that going up the Amazon would help in his quest! We explained. Meanwhile Emma, the youngest member of the group, who had come to support her mother, a patient, had produced a cunning device from the recesses of her clothing, and was tapping away on a keypad.

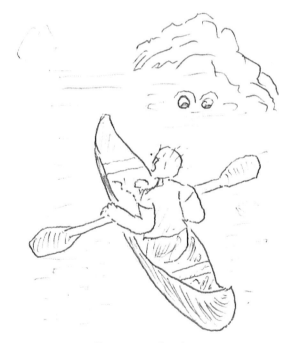

Going up the Amazon.

"I've found a copy! She announced. "Just one, held by such and such a bookshop, and priced at £24.50."

"Good heavens" exclaimed Tony. "I was expecting to have to pay double that for a copy."

I hope he has got the book by now, and it was a marvellous illustration of members of the group helping one another, across a pretty large generation and academic gap, I reckon!

This brings me on to one other very important result of being a cancer patient. Having seen at first hand how much help was given to me by the staff at my local hospital, and having also glimpsed how hard they worked, sometimes under considerable strain and stress, I also became aware of people working as volunteers in the oncology department. In fact I soon realised that there were volunteers, mainly older people of both sexes, working all over the hospital. I now know that there are over four hundred of them, and it is fair to say that our hospital would find it difficult to function without their help, especially in these days of funding deficits and staff cuts.

After my recovery from my first bout of cancer in 2004, I was recruited by our present Nurse Specialist Manager to work as a volunteer in the Cancer Information Centre, and the last five years have been some of the most fulfilling and rewarding of my life. The people I have been privileged to work with have been expert and dedicated, and the many patients I have met have been a true inspiration through their courage and kindness in the face of suffering and adversity.

I would very strongly suggest to those of you who are able to spare the time, to consider helping as volunteers at your local hospital. If you have had cancer yourself, you can bring a particular insight and empathy to your ministry, and complement those staff who have medical training. You will also have the privilege of working with a truly dedicated team, and doing a wonderfully worthwhile job.

CHAPTER 18. LASTING SYMPTOMS AND SUMMARY.

I can't pretend that having two bouts of cancer, apparently unrelated, in the last seven years, has been an enjoyable experience. The first one arrived completely out of the blue, when I should have said I had done everything possible in the realms of smoking, diet, drinking and exercise to avoid the disease. Unfortunately cancer does not work like that! The second one, seven years later, when I had been declared cured, was just as much of a shock, and possibly more so.

Looking back I have to be profoundly thankful for the facilities of my local hospital, doctor's surgery, and other support. The team at the hospital have not only nursed me, but have become friends over the years, and their expertise has been admirable. Then I have had the benefit of the most amazing modern equipment, in particular the three types of machines used to do scans, which have revolutionised diagnosis and the monitoring of patients. Again it is also the staff who operate and interpret these scans who do such a wonderful and lifesaving job for cancer patients.

And while we are in the mode of counting our blessings, let us also remember that all this is free, whereas in most countries in the world if developing cancer is not bad enough, it can also confront you with huge expense for treatment and medicines. Whatever the problems and challenges our N.H.S. and hospital trusts face, we are still incredibly lucky, which is another reason why being a volunteer is very necessary and rewarding. Most hospitals will have a department that deals with volunteers, and where you can make enquiries about helping in some way or another.

From a deep feeling of gratitude for what has been done for me, I can move on to assess my present situation, which will be not unlike that of many other cancer patients.

I do have lasting symptoms, and they are not likely to improve at my age, so I must learn to live with them! My first tumour, on my upper spine, has left me with a disabled left arm and hand. Very annoying, as I keep dropping things, but then at one point I could easily have been paralysed from the neck downwards, so I am indeed very fortunate. Then there is the Peripheral Neuropathy, which again leads to lack of sensation and clumsiness, as well as the problem of spelling the symptom!

My cancer produced heart problems, as has been the case for others, but I might easily have had these in any case, and without warning. In my case I have now been fitted with a pacemaker, and as long as I remember to wind it up I keep going very well!

I have a thyroid problem and a water retention problem, together with a blood pressure challenge, and that means five more tablets to consume with my porridge each day, or with my supper, and then I seem to be developing diabetes now, so that even a single grain of sugar has become a lovely dream from the past!

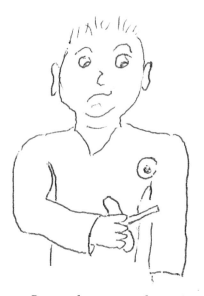

Remember to wind it up!

All in all I have to admit that I am not quite the man I was, and many of you will feel the same way. We just have to keep on taking the tablets!

That could be described as the negative side of the present situation. What about a more positive outlook?

I am still able to travel around my native East Anglia and lecture to a wide and fascinating variety of groups of people, who range from Church groups and fellowships to homemade wine makers. The latter meeting was a very convivial occasion, but I doubt whether the lovely audience remembered much that I had to say!

In the last seven years I have been able to travel further afield than ever before, - to South Island, New Zealand among many other places, and help with travel insurance and other medical matters has been available from my local hospital. I have been able to write, which I much enjoy, and I have even ventured into publishing, though whether that is wise in the present economic climate is an open question!

I can still do some physical work, in the garden or beyond, and walking and swimming continue to be the main means of keeping a reasonable level of fitness. Indoors I have films, music, painting, and various activities connected with my great hobby of Dissectology, - enthusiasm for jigsaw puzzles!

Having cancer myself, including an unlooked for refresher course, has meant that I can reach out to other cancer patients who are having a tough time, and even visit a few who live in my own area. The telephone remains a very good way of keeping in touch, and reminding people that they are not forgotten, even though their actual treatment has ended. I have not really mastered the art of texting as yet!

I hope that this small book will be another way of helping those who are fighting cancer, in one of its many forms, and I would again stress that every patient will have a different experience, but that asking for support is always a great help.

It has been intended that this book should be in every possible way a "signpost" book pointing the way to the many other sources of support for cancer patients. In the later chapters of this book we shall consider the role of carers, who can sometimes be left out of the equation, and who are enormously important. We shall also have contributions from other cancer support organisations, as well as from a N.H.S. General Practitioner.

We hope that the index will provide a quick means of finding what you want, and we suggest that you use the blank pages at the end of the book to note local information, the names of key people and their phone numbers. This will help to maximise the books usefulness, and make it your main reference point when you need information and support.

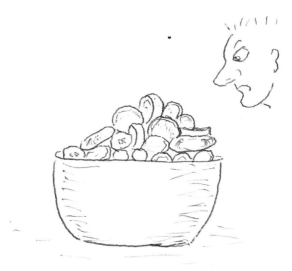

"Keep on taking the tablets."

CHAPTER 19. BEING THE CARER

There are probably as many 'reactions' to the news that one's partner / husband or wife / parent / relative or even worse ones' child has some form of cancer, as there are people who receive this news.

In some cases the news comes as a 'bolt out of the blue' – totally unexpected, in other cases it is the culmination of weeks or even months of investigations, ill-health and worry. Having experienced both scenarios I am not sure which is the hardest to cope with.

First and most importantly there is no 'Right' way to react. Some people react with tears and loud expressions of grief and need to talk endlessly about what has happened and what it means to them.

Some react with anger – directed at possibly the Drs, maybe their GP for perceived shortcomings and lack of urgency, maybe the Dr who broke the bad news with perceived lack of empathy or it may be some other healthcare professional. Sometimes the patient can receive some of the anger for life-style issues that might have contributed to the illness. And of course God often gets the blame –'Why has this happened to us?'

Other people find that they cannot talk about it at all – not to the patient or to anyone else.

All of these reactions and many in-between the two extremes do occur. The common factor for everyone is that they will need help in one form or another. There is no 'one size fits all' prescription for help. Carer's needs vary as widely as patients' needs. If one is caring for a parent, other relative or a friend it is different to caring for a partner or spouse. Everyone's previous experience is different too, so all carers need to be considered individually.

WHAT DOES THE DIAGNOSIS MEAN?

- *Is he/she going to die – now, soon, months or years? What is the expected outcome of the form of cancer that he/she has?* These are very difficult questions. Undoubtedly some types of cancer have much better outcomes than others. The present statistics are that more than 1 in 3 (42% recently reported) of us will get some form of cancer during our lifetime and that over 2 million people are living with it. It is best not to go straight to the Internet – there is a lot of 'miss-information' out there which can cause extra worry and stress. When you are given the diagnosis the chances that you will ask all the questions that you need answers to are very small – you keep thinking of more questions you want to ask while on the way home and in the days that follow. Don't be afraid to contact the hospital and ask if there is a Nurse Specialist that you can talk to. If there is a Cancer Information Centre – and many hospitals do have these now – go in and ask questions. Go and see your GP and talk to him/her, ask if there is a Macmillan Nurse you can talk to. The Macmillan Service has amalgamated with Cancer Bacup and produced a series of very good and accurate booklets covering all kinds of cancer and other related topics. Make a list of things you want to ask before your next hospital appointment. Never be afraid to ask questions. Nowadays Doctors are very open and honest with patients and relatives so you can feel reassured that you will be told what the situation is.

- *What sort of treatment is required? – will it be surgery alone or surgery + other treatment or will it be Chemotherapy or Radiotherapy or both? How long will the treatment last?* These questions should be discussed at the time of diagnosis though sometimes the specialists want to confer with colleagues before making firm decisions about the most appropriate treatment. For some forms of cancer there may be a choice of treatment and if this is the case the options will be carefully explained before a decision is made. The booklets explaining Chemotherapy and Radiotherapy which are produced by Macmillan are very helpful.
- *Will I/We be able to understand the medical information given to us by the Doctors and nurses? What do we do if we don't understand?* If you don't understand – Ask- and ask again if necessary! Most of us do not know much about cancer treatments until we are faced with the need for them. Doctors and nurses are usually very happy to explain in terms that lay people can understand. Nowadays Drs are given training in how to break bad news to people (thankfully the days of Sir Lancelot Spratt of the 'Doctor in the House' films are past history!) Again ask about talking to a specialist nurse at the hospital or a Macmillan nurse – these are found both in Oncology Departments in hospitals and out in the community.

- *Will I be able to cope – practically and emotionally?*
  'I've never wanted to be a nurse'! Most of us do find
  'hidden strength' to cope when the worst happens.
  Don't underestimate the effect of the shock of the
  diagnosis and be kind to yourself. You will probably
  have days when you feel that you can't cope. Everyone
  deals with these in different ways so try and work out
  what is best for you. It is often a help to get out of the
  house and away from the immediate worries. Some
  people find that physical exercise such as walking or
  swimming is a help or a game of golf for those who
  play. Others prefer to arrange to meet with a friend for a
  cup of tea or perhaps to go and see a film or do a bit of
  retail therapy! Just getting out for a short time can help
  restore one's perspective and help one to cope better.
- *What about the rest of the family – children,*
  grandchildren, parents, siblings? How do we talk to
  them about the diagnosis? It can be very hard telling
  the rest of the family the bad news. Sometimes the
  patient wants to do this themselves, others prefer to
  leave it to their partner, spouse or someone else.
  Prioritize who needs to be told – it can be very
  exhausting telling the story over and over again – I
  found that I could not manage more than two phone
  calls in an evening. Perhaps ask the closest family to
  contact other family members and friends – spread the
  load a bit. Don't worry if you find you cannot talk to
  people without getting emotional – they will understand
  and it is a very natural reaction. How you talk to
  children and grandchildren depends a great deal on their
  age and how much they can understand. Again there are

some helpful booklets which can be given to children to read or read to them. There is also information about what children can understand at different ages. Whatever their age children will sense that something is wrong so it is best to talk to them about it and try to give reassurance – lots of hugs and cuddles, they will cope better if they feel they are not being left out.

- *What about money? If it is the main breadwinner who is ill –how will we manage? Will I still be able to go out to work or will I need to be at home?* These are difficult questions and the situation will be different for every patient and carer. If the patient is still working it is obviously vital to talk to the employer – find out what the situation is with sick pay and whether flexible working is possible when and if the patient feels well enough. The same applies to the carer – it is important that people at work know what the situation is, most employers are sympathetic and as helpful as they are able to be. Benefit advice can be obtained – ask at the hospital and see if there are benefit advisors available. There are grants that can be obtained from Macmillan and other charities under certain circumstances. Don't be afraid to ask – if you don't ask you don't get!

- *What about hospital visits – for appointments, treatment and possibly in-patient stays? What about transport and costs?* The amount of time you have to spend at the hospital varies enormously. If surgery is required there will obviously be an in-patient stay. Sometimes Chemotherapy requires overnight stays –for the first dose or every time it is given. The regime of treatment will vary according to the form of cancer being treated. Radiotherapy is usually given as Out-patient treatment – sometimes 5 days a week for 6 weeks. There is more information about these treatments elsewhere in this book. It may be possible to get help with transport and parking costs and some hospitals have a hospital car service to help if there are problems. Again if you have difficulty getting to the hospital ask what help is available.

- *What can I do to help with the treatment – managing medications? Will injections be needed at home? If they are who will give them?* Managing medication can be a problem and often the patient does not feel able to do it themselves. A Dossett box which can be bought quite cheaply at the chemists can prove to be an invaluable tool. They have a 'drawer' for each day with up to 4 compartments. If there are multiple medications get a friend to sit with you when you fill it with the weeks' tablets. Often there are tablets to be taken immediately after treatment and then others to start a few days later. It requires quite a lot of concentration and to have someone to check it with is very reassuring! If daily injections are required it can be possible to arrange for the District Nurse to visit if the patient and carer feel they cannot do it themselves – don't feel guilty if this is something you just cannot do. It can be the last straw and you don't have to do it.
- *What about daily routines, diet, sleep?* Having a daily routine can be a help to many people but if you are not a 'routine' person don't feel you need to have one but do try to get medication taken on time. As far as diet is concerned there is more detailed advice within this

book. Try to have regular meals + snacks in between and most importantly eat well yourself even if the patient has little appetite. It is not the time to think about dieting or losing weight. Try and get enough sleep and rest yourself. If you share a double bed and the patient is restless you may need to think of twin beds or of sleeping in another room. Getting exhausted yourself will not help anyone.

- *Will the patient be able to lead a 'normal' life or will they be an invalid? Will we have to cancel holidays and other commitments?* Normal life versus being an invalid is another difficult question which depends on individual circumstances. It is a balance between being encouraging to keep life as normal as possible and being understanding when the patient feels exhausted and unwell. You won't get it right all the time – just do your best and ask advice from the professionals if necessary. Many treatment regimes go in cycles of 2,3 or 4 weeks. It can be worth keeping a diary of how the patient is feeling and coping as a pattern may easily emerge which enables you to plan activities at the best point in the cycle. We found this very helpful and planned visits out and friends to us at times when we were fairly sure that we would not need to cancel at the last minute. Holidays can be a problem – going abroad is not a good idea during a course of treatment and the hospital will almost certainly advise against it. You probably won't feel like going far from home but may enjoy a brief stay with relatives or friends or at a favourite place not too far from home. Go with how you both feel and there is life after treatment so look forward to a treat when the patient feels better.

- *What about the household / garden chores? How will I manage if he/she cannot do their share?* Accept any help offered! Try not to be too house or garden 'proud'. Prioritise what must be done and what can wait or be passed to someone else to do. It is not easy –most of us are fiercely independent but people do want to help and think what you would want to do if roles were reversed.

- *Do we need to make any alterations at home? Move a bed downstairs?* Don't do anything drastic in a hurry that you might regret later. You may need to have grab rails fitted in places to ensure safely, it should be possible to get help and advice with such things through the Occupational Therapy Dept either via the hospital or the community via your GP or other health care professional. Having a bed downstairs for day time resting might be a useful temporary measure.

- *How do I cope with the anxiety and added stress? How will I manage when he/she is possibly irritable and unreasonable when feeling unwell?* Being realistic the answer is probably 'with difficulty'! Having some 'time out' is probably essential. This may mean getting family or friends to come and 'patient sit' to allow you to get out. It is strange how even the need to go to the supermarket becomes a pleasure! If you don't have anyone who can help you ask about local voluntary groups such as Crossroads , these groups do often help with providing sitters. If the patient is really unwell and needs more expert help ask for a referral to the Marie Curie service which provides trained helpers.

Chemotherapy can often cause irritability even to those people who arc usually laid back and even tempered. If this does happen hold on to the knowledge that it will wear off after the chemotherapy is completed. Again just do your best – you won't get it right all the time – I certainly did not!

- *How can I find time for myself without causing resentment and without feeling guilty?* Looking after yourself is a vital part of caring for the patient. It will not help anyone if you get unwell. If you find that the patient appears resentful of your need for some 'space to yourself' talk to either someone in the team at the hospital or to your GP. It often helps if someone who is not emotionally involved can explain your needs to the patient in a calm way. Some people find that taking part in a Carers Group can help as you can talk to people who have similar problems and pick up tips and advice as well as support.

- *If I /We are not satisfied with aspects of care / treatment or worried about them who can we turn to for help?* The first thing to do is to talk to someone in the healthcare team who are looking after you, often things can be put right by sharing how you feel and why you are unhappy about your care. If this does not resolve the issue or if you feel unable to do this most hospitals have staff who are able to help you. Many hospitals have a PALS dept (Patient Advice and Liaison Service) who will talk to you and help you decide what action needs to be taken

Summary of tips and Hints for Survival

- LOOK AFTER YOURSELF! It is not 'selfish' to do this. If you as carer do not look after yourself and keep well then you will be unable to fulfill your role as carer and things really will fall apart at the seams.
- It is OK to feel angry / sad/ frustrated / stressed and any other negative feelings that you may have. Don't suppress these feelings, find someone to talk to and express them out loud. It is not just a cliché that 'a trouble shared is a trouble halved'.
- Make use of the professional support and help that is available. If you find the medical terminology daunting and hard to understand don't hesitate to ask for explanations. No-one is going to think that you are stupid or wasting their time.
- Some hospitals offer complementary therapies such as aromatherapy, reflexology and similar therapies to carers as well as to patients. If you are offered this Take it! If it is not mentioned ask if this is available.
- Accept help from family and friends with practical things – shopping / meals /laundry / ironing / cleaning / transport / patient-sitting to mention just e few! Basically accept any help that is going! It may be 'more blessed to give than to receive' but believe me it can be harder to accept help than give it – most of us like to think 'we can cope'! Remember that family and friends want to help and that you are helping them by allowing them to help you.

- Try to carry on with any hobbies or activities that you usually enjoy as far as possible. It is all part of looking after yourself. I personally find pottering in the greenhouse and garden very therapeutic and the fresh organic vegetables are a bonus!
- Exercise and fresh air are important. If you enjoy swimming or a few holes of golf or just a walk in the park or countryside all these things are beneficial. If there is a dog in the house the walking is an essential but I don't think that now is the time to get a dog for that reason alone!
- Finally DO NOT FEEL GUILTY when (not if) you are not as patient / loving / kind / understanding as you feel you ought to be! It is impossible to be an 'angel' all the time – if at all. YOU CAN'T GET IT RIGHT ALL THE TIME!

CHAPTER 20. SUPPORT FOR CANCER PATIENTS.

This next section of our book has been written to provide information on some of the additional means of help and support for cancer patients, and we are most grateful to the Health Care Professionals who have given of their time and expertise to help us all in this way.

The nature and amount of help available for patients and carers will vary from area to area of the U.K. and even more in different parts of the world. As has been stressed in this book, it is very much up to patients and carers to ask questions and seek information, using the starting points described in this book.

As we have explained, in the past cancer was regarded as the worst of all illnesses, and a diagnosis was considered to be the next thing to a death warrant. Thank goodness not only have treatment methods and diagnosis changed out of all recognition in our own lifetime, but attitudes have also changed in an amazing way.

One of the people who had a huge impact on this latter state of affairs was Dame Cicely Saunders, who founded St. Christopher's Hospice at Sydenham in the 1960s. Her vision was to see that all cancer patients who were terminally ill should be able to die in dignity, with their physical, medical and spiritual needs being catered for by specially trained doctors, nurses and chaplains.

As a result of her amazing ministry, death for cancer sufferers could be seen as a kind of triumph, rather than a defeat, and families and friends would feel a part of the patient's peaceful death. Today, Hospices are to be found all over the U.K. as well as in many other countries.

SPECIALIST PALLIATIVE CARE, - What is it?

Specialist Palliative Care Teams have historically supported patients with a cancer diagnosis. The focus of the team's work is to support a patient and the people close to them, usually family and friends. This care will be given during the patient's treatment, also at difficult times during the patient's illness, and as they approach the end of their lives. Specialist Palliative Care Teams may either be based in a hospital, or else in the community. Many such teams received initial funding from Macmillan Cancer Support, and are therefore known as Macmillan Teams, and the nurses that belong to such a team are designated Macmillan Nurses.

However, it has now been recognised that Specialist Palliative Care should not be confined to cancer patients alone, but should also be made available to patients with other chronic and progressive illnesses. Today Specialist Palliative Care Teams may be attached to a Hospice, which will provide the necessary funding. The Team may have a different name in such circumstances, but the service which is provided is the same. Here, at St. Elizabeth Hospice, our team is called the Community Clinical Nurse Specialist Team.

The Specialist Palliative Care Team provides specialist advice, support and information to patients and their families and friends. The team is able to:

Assess and manage difficult symptoms;

Provide emotional support and help deal with difficult fears and worries;

Help patients to determine future choices in terms of care;

Give practical advice regarding care, equipment and benefits:

The team can involve a large group of specialists, such as:

Occupational Therapists;
Physiotherapists;
Counsellors;
Chaplains;
Complementary Therapists,
Family Support workers;
Bereavement support Counsellors.

  The Specialist Palliative Care team works very closely with your own G.P., the District Nurses and the hospital team looking after a patient. Patients can receive specialist palliative care input in the hospital, in the community, at home or in a care home, a hospice or in hospital/community clinics.
  The focus of the team is to provide the most appropriate support for patients and their families in a wide variety of settings.

Friederike Englund,
Nurse Consultant,
St. Elizabeth Hospice,
Ipswich. U.K.

MACMILLAN CANCER SUPPORT.

History.

In 1911 Douglas Macmillan founded the "Society for the Prevention and Relief of Cancer" following his fathers death from cancer. His experience of the lack of existing services to support managing his fathers illness at home led to his founding of the Society.

Douglas wanted advice, information and support to be provided to all people with a diagnosis of cancer, together with the provision of nurses to attend to patients in their own homes, and this was the beginning of the present Macmillan Cancer Support service. Now, a hundred years later, Macmillan has founded 3,549 Clinical Nurse Specialist posts across the U.K. – both in hospitals and in the community.

Macmillan Clinical Nurse Specialists.

For many people affected by cancer, Macmillan nurses are a valued and trusted source of expert information, advice and support, and this is free of charge.

All Macmillan Nurses are registered nurses with a minimum of five years experience, and including at least two years in cancer care or palliative care. Each nurse completes specialist courses in managing pain or other symptoms of the illness, and also in psychological support for patients.

Macmillan nurses are usually employed by the N.H.S. and their posts are funded by Macmillan for a set time, - often the first three years. After that time, the long term funding is taken up by the N.H.S. or other partnership organizations, such as the local hospice. In East Suffolk, for example, the Community Macmillan Team is employed by St. Elizabeth Hospice.

How to get support from a Macmillan Clinical Nurse Specialist.

As a patient you will usually need to be referred by your G.P., Hospital Consultant, District Nurse or hospital staff. Macmillan nurses are available throughout most of the U.K. but if there is not a Macmillan Service in your local area, you can be referred to other alternative specialist services.

Within my own area, East Suffolk, referrals will be accepted from patients themselves, or their relatives (with the consent of the patient) as well as through health care professionals.
Here, referrals can also be made on line, via the St. Elizabeth Hospice website –www.stelizabethhospice.org.uk, and similar facilities will apply elsewhere. You can make referrals through the advice line, OneCall 0800 5670 111 or by faxing a referral form (which is available on the website) to your local hospice or Macmillan team.

Pauline Douglas.
Team Leader,
St. Elizabeth Community CNS,
Ipswich. U.K.

THE ROLE OF THE DISTRICT NURSING SERVICE IN THE CARE OF CANCER PATIENTS AT HOME.

Cancer services, and the way they are organised to support patients at home, can vary from area to area. In most cases the District Nursing service has a key role to play in providing direct care, with support and advice to patients, and their service is often the link with other professionals and agencies involved in care and treatment.

District Nurses work in teams, which are led by a sister, charge nurse or lead nurse, and may comprise qualified nurses and support workers, all of whom can be involved in supporting patients at home. District Nurses work closely with G.P.s and other members of the primary health care team, such as physiotherapists, occupational therapists, social workers and carers, as well as more specialist cancer services such as Macmillan nurses, Marie Curie nurses, oncology staff and hospice outreach services. Many doctor's surgeries have regular meetings specifically for the purpose of ensuring that all professionals involved with the care of cancer patients are working together, and the District Nurses are always included.

Although each service and specialist has their own role to play, this can sometimes become confusing for patients, and it is the District Nurses who usually liaise and coordinate things from the patient's perspective. They also undertake much of the clinical work when monitoring patients and helping to control any symptoms which they may have. The Nurses aim is to support patients who have to live with cancer, whilst helping them to maintain as much independence and quality of life as possible, and to enable them to stay at home for their treatment and care if that is what they wish.

District nursing teams may undertake an initial introductory visit to a patient following a diagnosis of cancer, to introduce themselves, answer any questions the patient or carer may have, and to provide helpful contact details. They may take blood tests or other samples as required or requested by the G.P. or hospital, and they may administer medication to help alleviate any pain or sickness that may result from the patient's condition or treatment. The District Nurses can also give advice on the type of medication, and will link closely with the G.P. and the pharmacist to ensure that the right kind of medication is prescribed, and they will respond to changes in the patient's condition as necessary. They will also advise on any continence issues or bowel care, involving other specialists if required. They will be involved in dressing wounds, and giving advice with regard to skin care if necessary. In general the District Nurses will support patients and their families, friends and carers with any issues or concerns that may arise.

District Nurses can also link with a range of care agencies and social services to ensure patients are supported with hygiene and personal care needs and have regular meals delivered if required. The District Nurses will work with social workers and other agencies to organize care workers to help with this aspect of patient care.

Many nursing teams also do assessments for equipment and aids to support patients at home. This can include adjustable height beds, commodes, walking aids, hoists and other relevant equipment, although in some areas they will link up with occupational therapists or physiotherapists who will order the necessary equipment.

The District Nurses will have a thorough understanding of how the patient's home area functions, and what is available to support you at home, as resources and services which are available vary from one area to another. They can also help you with advice on benefits and allowances, or else point you in the direction of an expert on these matters. The nurses are a vital source of information on many of the issues a patient may have not only with the clinical care they require, but also the many other factors that can arise such as how to source help around the house, find assistance with transport, and meet other people locally who are experiencing similar situations.

Care and support from the District Nurses is also available for those people who are caring for someone with cancer, and this can include linking with organizations and groups for those in a caring role, and continuing support after the death of a loved one.

The involvement of the District Nursing team can therefore be very varied, ranging from a telephone call asking for advice to regular visits to the patient's home, depending on what is required. Many patients get to know their nursing team very well during the period of their illness, and especially if the illness progresses, and they chose to die to home. In these circumstances the District Nurses will visit regularly to provide the necessary nursing care to facilitate this desire. The team are available to you and your family and friends from diagnosis onwards, in order to ensure that you all receive the care and support that you require.

Stacey-Anne Penny, District Nurse,
Community Team Lead,
Woodbridge Local Health Care Team,
Suffolk Community Healthcare.

THE ROLE OF THE GENERAL PRACTITIONER.

As a cancer patient you may encounter quite a few very expert specialists, but sometimes it is helpful to know that there is a generalist too; someone who can keep an eye on all the different aspects of your health and treatments.

Diagnosis.

It may be that your G.P. has been involved in the process of reaching your diagnosis of cancer, but sometimes the diagnosis is reached without any G.P. involvement (for example if the cancer was picked up as part of a screening programme.) Either way, your G.P. can discuss your diagnosis with you, and help you to understand what might need to happen next (tests, treatment etc).

Investigations.

Some investigations are simple (blood tests or x-rays, for example), but some can be more complex and it might be that you don't understand what the test is for, or what it involves. Your G.P. can be someone to talk to about this, who will know the answers to your questions.

Treatments and Medicines.

The majority of cancer treatments require the expertise of cancer specialists, and the teams in the hospital Oncology Department are very good at explaining the treatments in detail. A lot of treatments need to be done in the specialist clinics, but some medicines may be prescribed for you to take at home. The specialist clinics will usually start these prescriptions, and then will write to your G.P. to ask for further prescriptions if needed. If there is an urgent need for the specialist to ask the G.P. to do a prescription for you, they will fax or phone the G.P. and it will be ready as soon as needed. Other prescriptions may be less urgent, and most G.P. surgeries ask for 2-3 working days to get the prescription ready.

Symptom Management.

The specialist oncology clinics will give you a clear idea of what symptoms you may expect (for example possible side effects of treatment), and what can be done to help. There are some symptoms you may be given specific instructions about, asking you to contact the specialist clinic directly (for example developing a fever while on certain types of chemotherapy). If you are not sure about a particular symptom, your G.P. is a source of advice and can help with symptom management.

Co-ordinating with different services.

There are quite a few different services available to help with the management of cancer: oncologists, radiotherapists, Macmillan Cancer Support nurses, specialist oncology nurses, Community Nurses, Hospice Services including Hospice at Home, Marie Curie nurses, CRUSE bereavement counselling and many others. Your G.P. can help direct you to whatever service is needed, co-ordinating between services, and will also be a common point of reference as most correspondence about your care will be copied to your G.P.

Dr. Jonathan Knight.
Lattice Barn Surgery,
Ipswich. Suffolk.

HOW MARIE CURIE CANCER CARE CAN HELP YOU.

Established in 1948, the same year as the N.H.S., Marie Curie Cancer Care is a U.K. charity dedicated to the care of people with terminal cancer and other life-limiting illnesses. Our services are always free for patients and their families.

We have more than 2,000 Marie Curie Nurses and Healthcare Assistants across the U.K., providing end of life care for patients at home, and support for their families.

There are nine Marie Curie Hospices across the U.K. offering specialist care for in-patients, along with day services. We also conduct palliative care research to find better ways of caring for terminally ill people.

Here, in Suffolk, U.K., our team of Marie Curie Nurses provide an overnight service to care for patients with end of life care needs at home or in a care home. In addition, we have two Marie Curie discharge liaison nurses working at the local hospitals to help patients to get discharged home safely and comfortably, and to ensure that they have the appropriate care and support after their discharge.

You should talk to your district nurse or community matron to see if they think you could benefit from Marie Curie's services. They will refer you to our service if they think it is suitable for you.

FURTHER INFORMATION.

Visit Marie Curie's Website for Film Guides featuring practical demonstrations focusing on personal care and everyday living.

As well as films, you will find our website is packed with information for people with cancer, and other life-limiting illnesses, as well as for their families.
www.mariecurie.org.uk

Our address is; Marie Curie Cancer Care,
89 Albert Embankment, London SE1 7TP.
Free call Helpline: 0800 716 146.

Support Marie Curie Cancer Care.

Our services are free to patients and their families, but we rely on the generous support of the public to continue our work. Please visit our website to find out more
www.mariecurie.org.uk
or phone us on 0800 716 146. (Free call.)

Sue Hughes,
Marie Curie Nursing Sister.

SIGNPOST TO USEFUL CONTACTS.

There is a great deal of very helpful information for cancer patients now available, in booklet form, on line, and on the telephone. Local information centres can be an ideal starting place, as you can talk to an expert and detail your personal requirements.

Macmillan Cancer Support, as already stated, offer a large variety of helpful advice, with many booklets. Their Helpline, on 0808 808 0000 throughout the U.K. is available during the working day. Calls are free.

The Macmillan booklet "Cancer Survivors Guide" is a very good and comprehensive mine of information, and can be obtained from Macmillan Cancer Support, 89 Albert Embankment, London SE1 7UQ or at www.macmillam.org.uk

There are organizations which cater for patients with a particular cancer. Examples are:

Bowel Cancer U.K. 7 Rickett St. London SW6 1RU.
Helpline: 0870 850 6050
Brain Tumour U.K. Tower House, Latimer Park,
Chesham, Bucks. HP5 1TU. Helpline; 0845 4500 386
Breast Cancer Care, Kiln House, 210 New Kings Road,
London SW6 4NZ. Helpline: 0808 800 6000.
British Red Cross. 44 Moorfields, London, EC2Y 9AL.
Telephone 0844 871 1111.
Carers U.K. 20 Great Dover St. London. SE1 4LX.
Carers Line 0808 808 7777
Kids Cancer Charity (Christian Lewis Trust.) 62 Walter
Road, Swansea. SA1 4PT. Tel: 01792 480500.

CLIC Sargent. Horatio House, 77-85 Fulham Palace Road, London W6 8JA. Tel: 020 8752 2800.

Lymphoedema Support Network, St. Lukes's Crypt. Sydney Street, London SW3 6NH. 020 7351 4480

Lymphoma Association. P.O.Box 386. Aylesbury, Bucks. HP20 2GA. Helpline 0808 808 5555

Myeloma U.K. Broughton House, 31 Dunedin Street, Edinburgh, EH7 4JG. Tel: 0800 980 3332

Oesophageal Patients Association. 22 Vulcan House, Vulcan Rd. Solihull. B91 2JY. Tel: 0121 704 9860.

Pancreatic Cancer U.K. 3rd Floor, Market Towers, 1 Nine Elms Lane, London SW8 5NQ. Tel: 0118 947 2934.

Prostate Cancer Charity. 1st Floor, Cambridge House, 100 Cambridge Grove, Hammersmith. W6 0LE. Helpline: 0800 074 8383.

Roy Castle Lung Cancer Foundation. Enterprise Way, Wavertree Technical Park, Liverpool. L13 1FB. Helpline: 0800 358 7200

If you can't find the information or booklet you want, keep on asking until you have it!

INDEX.

USEFUL TELEPHONE
    NUMBERS

DATES TO REMEMBER

NOTES

NOTES